GUIDE FOR TRAINEES
IN
GENERAL PRACTICE

GH00976171

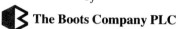

GUIDE FOR TRAINEES
IN
GENERAL PRACTICE

Edited by John Fry

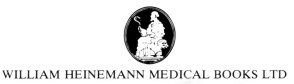

WILLIAM HEINEMANN MEDICAL BOOKS LTD

Heinemann Medical Books Limited
23 Bedford Square, London WC1B 3HH

First published 1982
Reprinted 1983, 1986

ISBN 0-433-10917-3

Typeset by Preface Ltd, Salisbury, Wilts.
Printed in Great Britain by J. W. Arrowsmith Ltd, Bristol.

CONTENTS

PREFACE

Working in general practice after the seclusion and protection of hospital work is a novelty and a revelation to most trainees. General practice is a special field of medical care with its own methods and techniques and its own diseases and problems. For the first time the young doctor will be faced with packages of unstructured medical, social, family and personal problems all rolled into a single consultation.

Vocational training aims to bridge the gaps (or gulfs) between general practice and hospital work. To help the trainee this guide has been prepared, based on our combined joint experience of over 100 practice years in our varied practices and on many years of teaching trainees.

Who is this book for? Primarily it has been written for the trainee but, of course, trainers should study it too if they are to be able to anticipate questions and cover the curriculum.

Why has it been written? Because we believe there is need for a simple, practical, clear and short book for trainees to guide them during their training period and after.

What is in it? There are three parts:
- Part I deals with the important matters of organisation and administration.
- Part II sets investigation and management of patients in a general practice perspective emphasising the practical differences from hospital work.
- Part III looks beyond the training period and seeks to alert the young practitioner on issues to be considered in choosing a practice.

We have enjoyed writing this book and learnt much while doing so. In dedicating it to future generations of trainees and trainers we hope their enjoyment and instruction while using it will be as great as our own.

We thank Richard Emery, Dr Richard Barling and Pat Pembroke of William Heinemann Medical Books for their encouragement and help.

1982   John Fry,
                                                                    Beckenham.

LIST OF CONTRIBUTORS

Five general practitioner teachers

- John Fry, Beckenham, Kent.
- Eric Gambrill, Crawley, Sussex.
- Peter Martin, Basildon, Essex.
- Alistair Moulds, Basildon, Essex.
- Gillian Strube, Crawley, Sussex.

PART I
ADMINISTRATION AND ORGANISATION

1. THE NATURE OF GENERAL PRACTICE AND THE WORK OF THE PRACTICE

General practice, or primary care, is an essential and inevitable aspect of medical care in all countries. Sandwiched between self-care by individuals and families and specialist services in local hospitals, general practice serves as the first point medical contact for the public, except for some accidents and emergencies which may go direct to casualty departments.

Special Features of General Practice

Direct access. Patients may consult the family doctor when they think it is necessary. Specialists can be seen by referral only.

Local availability. Practice premises have to be reasonably accessable to the patients. Elderly patients and young mothers have to be able to get there easily, though most patients are now more mobile than before.

The presentation of illnesses. Patients bring vague collections of symptoms that have to be assessed, diagnosed and managed, or at least arranged into a reasonably defined clinical package, before referral to a specialist. First contact care demands skill, knowledge, understanding and experience.

The small community. The population base of one general practitioner is about 2500 patients, whereas the district general hospital provides services for about 250 000. Between 5 and 10% of these patients may move in any one year.

Continuing care. As the population is fairly static, patients and doctors can get to know each other well. Patients have to be managed through many different acute or chronic, physical or emotional conditions and it is this continuing care that is the hallmark of British general practice. This is in contrast to the transient and episodic nature of the care given in hospitals.

The incidence of diseases. If the GP has 2500 patients and the local hospital covers 250 000 then the GP will see only 1/100 of hospital-type diseases. Thus the GP will diagnose 3–5 cases of acute appendicitis a year while the local surgical units will operate on 300–500. The common diseases of general practice are, in order:

respiratory infections, skin disorders, psychosocial problems, gastro-intestinal disturbances and rheumatism.

Under the NHS each person is entitled to care from a general practitioner. In addition to serving as the basis for remuneration by capitation fees, registration of each patient also provides continuity of clinical records that are passed from one practitioner to the next. This may also be used to construct an age–sex register to give a statistical picture of the population at risk.

Work of the Practice

The bulk of the work is done in consultations at the surgery and during home visits. The GP also spends a considerable amount of time doing routine immunisations, examinations, repeat prescriptions, writing reports, administration and work outside the practice.

Consultation

About 80% of face-to-face contacts with patients occur in consultations in the practice premises.

Purpose of the consultation

- Usually regarded as the opportunity for the patient to seek the doctor's advice and support, it provides first contact care for new problems and continuing care for chronic problems through repeat attendances.
- The consultation may also be used to allow the patient to ventilate feeling and emotions. It may be an opportunity to manipulate others, an activity that is not confined to patients.
- Teaching is an important part of the consultation and this is probably the most effective method of health education.
- Do not forget the value of the general social chat during which a lot of information about the patient and the family may be obtained.

Conducting the consultation

The history. This is the most important part of the consultation. The GP gleans information about the patient over many consultations and the formal type of history-taking has to be modified to suit the short general practice consultation. Trained to take a history on the basis of questions and answers, the GP should also be aware that more useful information can sometimes be obtained by allowing the patient time to express feelings and fears.

The examination. Should be selective rather than comprehensive, but mistakes will be made if a necessary examination is skimped. Take the opportunity to record vital indices, such as blood pressure, weight and urine analyses.

The action. Explanation of the diagnosis and pathology in clear and simple terms is vital. This is necessary if you expect the patient to undertake some self-care and self-observation. Investigations have to be organised but only where they are strictly relevant and necessary.

Treatment. May just be a prescription, but may also consist of advice about lifestyle, rest, work and many other matters.

Appointment systems

An appointment system benefits patients and doctors by saving waiting times and in affording a better distribution of work. This is true only if the system runs fairly and is not used merely as an attempt to limit patient demand.

Appointment systems are particularly useful for increasing compliance for immunisation and checks on diabetes, blood pressure, etc.

Home visits

Home visiting is still a vital part of British general practice, though it is much less frequent than in the past. More families are mobile, wait in the surgery for a shorter time and GPs are not as competitive as they were. Many GPs also delegate much of the chronic sick visiting to nurses.

The value of home visits

(1) The doctor is given the privilege of entering the patient's home and much can be observed about the standard of living and social attitudes.

(2) The needs of the elderly for aids or structural alterations may be assessed.

(3) Home visits do help to develop better doctor/patient relationships provided that the doctor does not see the request as demanding or manipulative.

Disadvantages

(1) Home visits are more time-consuming than surgery consultations.

(2) The doctor may feel less in command through not being on his or her home ground (not always a bad thing).

(3) Lack of surgery facilities for doing speculum examinations, proctoscopy, etc.

(4) Commonest complaint against GPs is for non-visiting.

The telephone

The telephone is a double-edged sword. The usual method of communication between patient and doctor in emergencies, it is being increasingly used by patients to obtain routine advice and information and to order repeat prescriptions. As more patients have telephones installed in their homes, so the traffic of calls into the surgery increases. A readily available telephone also tends to lower the anxiety threshold needed to initiate a call for help.

The telephone is useful for:

(1) giving advice about minor problems;

(2) taking messages for prescriptions, thereby avoiding the need for patients to travel and reducing congestion in the practice premises; and

(3) giving patients the results of tests and other information.

Telephone technique

- A kind considerate manner helps the interaction to proceed smoothly.
- If the patient perceives the doctor as well-meaning then the doctor's advice is more likely to be accepted.

- Patients who are very anxious are likely to be aggressive on the telephone. Patiently sort out the problem first: remonstrate later.
- Avoid direct refusals when requests for visits are made. Discuss the indications but leave the final decision to the caller. Educate as necessary later.

Repeat prescribing and prescribing for the unseen patient

About half of all prescriptions are written for 'unseen patients'. These are mostly repeats but often they are issued in response to a telephone request for help.

Precautions

(1) Be very careful if you prescribe for an unseen patient. If it is a minor illness—is a drug necessary? If the illness is bad enough to demand a drug—should the patient not be seen?

(2) A note of all prescriptions issued should be made.

(3) Repeat prescribing is made easier and more accurate if the patient is issued with a prescription card.

(4) There must be some system for making sure that patients on long-term therapy are reviewed at regular intervals

Out of hours cover

Although the NHS contract specifies 24-hour responsibility it is generally recognised that continuous cover is impossible for most doctors. Even so, the GP is responsible for making sure that there is medical cover when he is not available.

Organisation

- Single-handed practitioners or small groups may make reciprocal arrangements with neighbouring practices.
- Larger groups may organise in-practice rotas.
- Commercial deputising services employ doctors to provide cover and charge appropriate fees. In some areas doctors have organised deputising services on a cooperative basis.
- The main disadvantage of deputising services is that unfamiliar doctors see your patients and they may have very different ideas from yours about the management of some illnesses.

Work outside the practice

Roughly two out of three GPs have regular employment outside their practices.

Varieties of work

- They may have hospital appointments or practise privately.
- They may teach or write.
- They may be medical officers to schools, industry, homes, clubs, or voluntary organisations.
- They may be undertaking medical examinations for insurance, government agencies, or sport groups.

2. PREPARING FOR PRACTICE

Choosing a Training Practice

In some areas trainees are now allocated to a specific practice but generally trainers and trainees are allowed to go through a process of mutual selection. Choose the area in which you do your traineeship carefully, because you are likely to find your permanent job in the same area.

Characteristics of a good training practice

- The practice does not depend on the trainee to fulfil service commitments.
- All the partners are interested in the training.
- The practice should be busy enough to give good experience.
- Organisation should allow enough time for teaching.
- The trainer should have a clear plan for the year but should be flexible enough to negotiate details with you.

Before deciding on a practice, talk to as many trainees and trainers as you can. You will get much useful information this way.

Contracts and conditions

There are no set rules about hours or conditions of work, which are a matter for negotiation between you and your trainer, but remember:

(1) get a contract *before* you start work;

(2) model contracts are available from the British Medical Association (BMA);

(3) make sure you know what the hours of work are and what the out-of-hours commitments are; and

(4) leave entitlements are usually the same as those of senior house officers but may be less if the partners in the practice take less time off.

The trainee's duties

The trainer will probably specify in the contract that:

(1) the trainee will diligently apply himself/herself to work and educational activities as directed by the trainer;

(2) the trainee will not undertake outside professional duties;

(3) all fees earned by the trainee belong to the practice;

(4) suitable transport will be provided by the trainee; and

(5) membership of a defence organisation is compulsory.

Tools and equipment

Most contracts specify that the trainer is responsible for providing equipment. Nevertheless, most doctors like to have their own basic tools.

- A visiting bag and contents.
- Two stethoscopes—one for the bag, one for the surgery.
- A small ophthalmoscope-auroscope set.

Do not spend too much money at this stage because it is not tax deductible until you are self-employed.

Responsibilities

Although he/she is employed by the trainer, the trainee is a registered practitioner and is therefore responsible for clinical mishaps. The trainer as the employer may also be implicated.

It is in your own interests to do a fair share of the normal work of the practice so that you gain adequate experience during the year.

Remuneration

Details are in the statement of fees and allowances—the Red Book issued by the DHSS, containing all regulations and sales of payment for doctors—(make sure you read it).

Salary is related to the last NHS hospital post held. Payment is increased on the incremental date to next point in the scale.

Removal expenses may be paid. If in doubt contact the finance officer at the Family Practitioner Committee (FPC).

Other earnings. By regulation, the trainer cannot make any extra payments.

All fees normally belong to the practice.

Part-time work in off-duty hours. To do this, you must get the permission of the trainer *and the FPC*.

Telephone. The cost of installing a new telephone or a bedside extension is reimbursable by the FPC.

Car allowance is not automatically tax deductible and must be declared to the tax inspector.

Excess rent. Look up the Red Book or ask the FPC for details.

Interview expenses. Expenses for an interview with a trainer are payable by the responsible FPC provided that an offered job is not refused without good reason.

Sickness. Salary will be paid for up to three months. If the trainee is away for more than two weeks the training period will be extended to compensate for this.

Maternity leave. To be eligible, the trainee must have completed at least 12 months of NHS service immediately before the application. For details see the Red Book.

3. MEDICAL RECORDS

The general practitioner NHS medical records are unique in that they provide a life-long account of the patient's medical history. Virtually all the present stock of records are in the old Lloyd George envelopes because only a few general practitioners have been able to convert to A4-size records. The potential usefulness of the records as a clinical, teaching or research tool is often marred by the fact that information, if recorded at all, may be haphazard or illegible. Information retrieval is often laborious or impossible.

Reasons for good record-keeping

- To refresh your memory about your patient's history.
- To help other doctors who may see your patient.
- For medicolegal purposes.
- Research projects need accurate clinical information.
- Good records are useful tools in teaching sessions.
- Almost any audit process depends on accurate notes.

Characteristics of good records

(1) All episodes are recorded legibly.
(2) Ideally each episode should have the following recorded.
   S. Subjective. Patients complaints and observations.
   O. Objective. Examination and investigations.
   A. Analysis. Concise summary of position.
   P. Plan. Plan of action
(3) Records should contain a data base with information about family history, past and present problems, social history, allergies, immunisation status, etc.
(4) The necessary information is easily retrievable.

How to achieve the ideals of good records

- All hospital letters and continuation cards should be secured in chronological order.
- Use a standard format for recording episodes. You can use the mnemonic given above (that is SOAP) or invent your own.
- The data base. Make a point of recording occupation, marital status, etc., on the envelope. Some doctors keep the back of the envelope for notes on immunisation and other indices. Some practices have a special data base card which can be filled in bit by bit or patients can be asked to fill in a questionnaire—easiest when they first join the practice.
- *Summary*. Once the volume of a record envelope gets beyond a certain point it becomes progressively more difficult to extract information quickly. A summary of major events on a separate card is helpful. Once this has been done the thick files may be filleted. Only the key letters and pathology forms need be retained.

Records to facilitate continuous care

Most illnesses needing continuous care require the doctor to do routine checks—for example, diabetics should have their fundi looked at once a year. This process is made easier if special cards are used. The universally accepted example of this is the antenatal cooperation card. Similar cards have been designed for diabetes, hypertension and family planning.

Repeat prescribing may also be better controlled if patients on regular medication have their details recorded on special cards which also note the number of prescriptions issued and when the patient should be seen next.

Research registers

These are simply files of information about patients which allow easy abstraction of statistical and other information.

Age–sex register

The age–sex register is the basic register for any type of statistical research work. It can also be used to identify certain groups for surveillance—for example, cervical smears for women over 35.

Disease registers

These are lists of patients with certain illnesses. The numbers recorded will be as large or as small as the doctor's interests dictate. Useful as a quick way to identify groups of patients with certain illnesses for research, audit or teaching purposes.

The A4 record

A large file to take A4 sheets. Theoretically the larger format should help the doctor to maintain useful and tidy notes. However, the larger size does not ensure good records (remember what most hospital files look like).

Advantages

- More space for recording details.

- Larger format should make them tidier.
- Hospital letters and forms may be filed flat.

Disadvantages
- Can just become large untidy notes
- More space needed—more cabinets—bigger rooms.
- Cost of conversion can be quite high.

Family records

Some practices file all the records of the members of a family together. Useful if you wish to refer to the others during a consultation.

Computers

A few practices are beginning to use computers for various aspects of medical record-keeping. Mini-computers are particularly suitable for age, sex and disease registers. Extracting information is quick and easy. Clinical records need complicated equipment that would cost too much for most general practitioners. However, some pioneer units at Exeter, Hackney and elsewhere are developing systems for use in general practice.

Confidentiality

The general practitioner should make sure that his records remain confidential. They should be locked up when not in use and the staff should be given access only on an essential-user basis.

4 CERTIFICATES

Issuing certificates is an essential though not always enjoyable part of the general practitioner's job. When you sign one you are putting the authority of your profession behind it. Never do this unless you are sure of the facts and that it is justified. You may often be pressed to give certificates without seeing the patient or on tenuous grounds. Do not give in to emotional or financial persuasion.

False certification is an offence that can be reported to the General Medical Council (GMC). In most years one or two doctors are disciplined for this—so beware.

NHS Certificates

The GP is obliged by his terms of service to issue certificates without payment to patients who are entitled to them.

Sickness

Patients are entitled to certificates if they have been or are likely to be off work for a week or longer and if they pay a full stamp or have an industrial disease.

Form Med. 3

The usual certificate for sickness. Used for insurance purposes only, and the patient must be seen. At the back of the pad there are forms for requesting the regional medical officer to give an opinion about the patient's fitness for work. You must also notify him if you have used a false diagnosis on the certificate.

Form Med. 5

For use retrospectively or when the patient has not been seen but is under hospital care.

Maternity

These certificates enable expectant mothers to claim the various benefits to which they are entitled.

Form FW8

Issued at the start of the pregnancy. To claim free prescriptions, dental treatment, etc.

Mat. B1

Issued after the 26th week. Claims maternity grant and allowance.

Private Certificates

A doctor is not obliged to issue these. The BMA issue lists of recommended fees. Private certificates should not be issued any more casually than NHS ones.

Reports

Employers, insurance companies, solicitors and many other agencies may approach the general practitioner for reports on patients.

(1) Make sure the patient gives consent in writing.
(2) Draw the attention of the patient to any detrimental information you have before you make the report.
(3) Reports should go direct to another professional—a solicitor, for example.
(4) Be sure of your facts. You may be questioned about them in court.

Death Certificates

It is a statutory obligation to issue a death certificate.

- Write clearly and make sure of your facts.
- There is no legal necessity to visit after death, but it is kind and advisable to do so.
- Do not issue a certificate if patient was not seen within 2 weeks of death or if you have any doubt about the nature of the death (*see* pp. 28, 119). Read the instructions in the front of the book of certificates.

Cremation Certificates

Part I

Normally given by the doctor issuing the death certificate. The body must be seen and examined.

Part II

Given by an independent doctor of at least 5 years' standing who should question the patient's doctor and relatives or nurses. You must see and examine the body.

5. THE PRACTICE TEAM

The practice team is a relatively new concept. General practitioners used to work in isolation (and some still do). There has been a progressive trend towards the development of group practices and the employment of ancillary staff such as secretaries and receptionists. In many areas primary care in the community is now a team effort.

There are advantages and disadvantages to team work.

Advantages

- Improving communication
- Dissemination of knowledge.
- Maximum use of specialist skills.
- Sharing of responsibility.
- Understanding the work of others.

Disadvantages

- Personality clashes and status problems.
- Shelving or dodging responsibility.
- Patient may not know whom to relate to.
- A big team needs organisation.
- Time needed for meetings.

Composition of the team

(1) The GPs and the staff employed by them; and
(2) Staff employed by the Health Authority.

Health Authority Staff

These are community workers who may cover a geographical area or who may be attached to a GP. They are primarily responsible to the health authority and GPs and therefore have to work with them rather than over them.

District nurses.
Health visitors.
Midwives.
Social workers (who are actually employed by the local authority).

District nurses

- They are state registered nurses (SRNs) usually with special training, who do home nursing.
- In some areas they are allowed to work in surgeries.
- They may be assisted by state enrolled nurses (SENs) or unqualified bath assistants.
- Good relationships are essential because the district nurse will be looking after most of the chronically sick patients in the practice,
- They are experts in obtaining sick room equipment, night sitters, and other aids.

Health visitors

- They are SRNs who also have at least part I of the midwifery certificate.
- Further training is necessary to obtain the health visitors' certificate.
- Their work is directed by the community nursing officer.
- They are obliged to visit all newborn babies as soon as possible after the midwife stops attending.
- A major part of their work is the supervision of children in the community. Regular assessment of developing children with the objective of detecting physical, social or mental handicaps takes up much of their time.
- They may also undertake health education, run relaxation and mothercraft classes, and give counselling to families with social and emotional difficulties.
- Mothers use health visitors for advice about all sorts of problems and much of their work overlaps that of social workers.

Midwives

- Midwives are SRNs who go on to obtain parts I and II of the midwifery certificate.
- Their work includes making sure that home conditions are suitable for confinements or for early discharge from hospital; undertaking deliveries in the home or in GP obstetric units; and doing antenatal care either in the GPs surgery or on their own.

17

Social workers

- Most social workers are in teams allocated to a geographical area. Very few are attached to GPs.
- Relationships are much better if you get to know your local social workers and make sure that they can contact you when necessary.
- Their main statutory duty is the supervision of the welfare of children in the community.
- They also undertake the community care of: the mentally handicapped; the physically handicapped; the elderly; people with social or emotional problems; and the mentally ill.

Staff Employed by the GP

Telephonists, receptionists and secretaries

In small practices the staff may have to fulfil all these functions. In larger units they may specialise. Receptionists have a vital role in the practice. Usually the point of first contact, so a kind efficient response from them is essential.

Receptionist work

The work of receptionists may include the following.

Appointments. Keeping the doctor and the patients happy.
Visits. Taking messages for visits. Trying to match expectations of patients and views of the GP.
Prescriptions. Taking messages and filling in the FP 10s as directed.
Forms. Registering new patients. Dealing with claim forms for item-of-service fees.
Surgery. Running surgery session smoothly. Keeping doctor to time tactfully.
Records. Getting records in and out of the files. Tidying up records and filing letters.
Advice. Giving simple advice about other services, welfare foods, clinics, etc.

Make sure that the staff doing a responsible job get adequate training and remuneration. Give clear instructions and regularly discuss problems with them.

18

The practice manager

Discovering the joys of delegation, more GPs are appointing managers. They may be full-time or part-time depending on the size of the practice and the work delegated.

The main functions are as follows:

Staff Management. Dealing with training, wages, tax and problems.
Stock Control. Obtaining drugs, dressings, stationery.
Maintenance. Organising cleaning, repairs, decorating.
The FPC. Dealing with forms, claims, records.
Accounts. Keeping the practice books.
Initial management of patient complaints and problems.

Nurses

An increasing number of GPs are employing their own nurses because it is easier to direct their work and to make it fit in with the surgery hours. Most of them are employed in treatment rooms. Their functions are:

- Nursing procedures, dressings, injections.
- Dealing with pathology specimens, taking blood and urine samples.
- Handling stock control of drugs.
- Giving advice about simple illnesses.
- Assisting at minor operations, fitting intrauterine contraceptive devices.
- Undertaking electrocardiograms (ECGs).
- Undertaking immunisation.

Some doctors are offering nurses of suitable calibre further training to extend the scope of their work. They may then undertake the following duties:

- Routine follow-up of chronic illnesses such as hypertension, diabetes and obesity.
- Visiting the housebound.
- Family planning advice, repeat pills, caps.
- Cervical smears.
- First visits for simple illnesses like chickenpox.
- Special investigations, ECGs and allergy tests.

Whatever role is delegated to the nurse, the GP has the responsibility of ensuring that the nurse is adequately trained and that she agrees to the delegation.

The GP as an Employer

Like many other employers, the GP must comply with the Employment Acts. Employees must have proper job description, a contract, comfortable and safe conditions of work. National insurance and tax deductions must be made. Seventy per cent of the salaries of up to two full-time staff per partner may be reclaimed from the Family Practitioners Committee (FPC), claims being made each quarter on form RAN1.

Health Centres

In most centres staff are employed direct by the health authority, 30% of the cost then being reclaimed from the GPs (in a few health centres the GPs are allowed to hire their own staff).

Advantages

GPs are relieved of the tasks of hiring and firing. No work concerned with wages, tax, etc:

Disadvantages

Staff are tied to pay scales that are sometimes inadequate. The system is often inflexible.

The GP Members of the Team

The general practitioner is an independent businessman who contracts with the FPC to provide a primary medical service for the patients on the practice list. As from the 16th August 1982 all principals entering general practice will have to be vocationally trained for 3 years or to have had equivalent experience approved by the Joint Committee on Postgraduate Training (JCPT).

A suitably trained doctor may enter practice in the following ways.

(1) By joining an established partnership.

(2) By applying for a vacancy advertised by an FPC.
(3) By setting up in practice in an open or a designated area.
In a designated area an initial practice allowance may be payable.

Finance

The practice is paid a basic practice allowance for each partner.
Capitation and item of service fees are then added as appropriate.

There are special allowances for seniority, vocational training and
designated areas. All the details are in the Statement of Fees and
Allowances (SFA); make sure you get a copy and read it.

Partners divide the income according to the practice agreement.
The only regulation is that the lowest paid partner must not earn
less than one-third the share of the highest paid one.

Contracts

Like any other business arrangement the partnership should be
regulated by a carefully drafted contract. The characteristics of a
good partnership are:

(1) There should be an equitable distribution of income.
(2) Adequate provision should be made for sickness, maternity
leave, etc.
(3) Decisions should be taken democratically.
(4) Partners should be encouraged to develop new ideas and
interests.
(5) Regular meetings should be held to discuss administration
and clinical practice.

Assistants

Some practices employ an assistant rather than take on a new partner.

● The relationship is that of employee to employer.
● The FPC does make a payment for an assistant but this is less
than the basic practice allowance for a partner.

Trainers

To be a trainer the GP has to be appointed by the GP sub-committee of the regional postgraduate committee. The criteria for selection vary from region to region but usually include:

(1) At least three years in practice;
(2) Good references;
(3) Premises, records and facilities must pass inspection by the regional adviser;
(4) The GP has attended a trainer's course; and
(5) He or she takes an active part in local workshops and post-graduate meetings.

The trainer has to submit himself or herself to reselection at regular intervals.

Locums

Locums are necessary in small practices to maintain a service during leave and sickness absences.

- The GP is responsible for finding locums and for making sure that they are competent.
- If the locum is in breach of the terms of service the GP is responsible.
- In certain circumstances the FPC will pay part of the cost of a locum.

6. RELATIONSHIPS WITH OTHERS

Vocational Training

The Joint Committee on Postgraduate Training (JCPT)

The overall supervision and the issuing of certificates are the responsibility of the JCPT. The committee is formed by representatives of the General Medical Services Committee (GMSC) and the Royal College of General Practitioners (RCGP) and is housed at the College headquarters at Prince's Gate, London SW7 1PU.

The JCPT sends teams of visitors to inspect the various vocational training schemes at regular intervals.

The postgraduate deans

The deans are based in the local university and are responsible for postgraduate education in the region. They supervise the work of the various postgraduate institutes and the clinical tutors in the postgraduate centres.

The GP regional advisers.

The advisers are on the staff of the postgraduate deans and they are university employees. They are GPs with extensive experience of training.

Their remit is the day-to-day supervision of courses and trainers, but they are also concerned with GP continuing education.

Vocational training course organisers

These are local GPs who organise the half-day release course and the rotating hospital jobs for the three-year trainees. They help and supervise the work of local trainers.

If you have problems

You should first ask your trainer or local course organiser but if you do not wish to discuss the matter at local level, speak to your regional adviser. The secretary in the postgraduate centre should be able to supply the name and address.

The Structure of Vocational Training

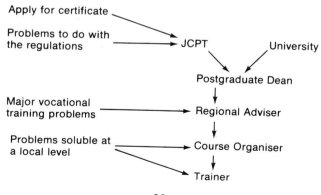

Patients and Families

Enjoyable and successful general practice depends on maintaining a good long-term relationship with patients. Friendliness has to be combined with firm management and this calls for a considerable amount of skill. The essential features of a good GP/patient relationship are as follows.

Mutual respect

The patient must respect the doctor as a person and as medical technician. The doctor has to earn this respect.

The doctor must also recognise the fact that patients have an importance and a dignity of their own.

Remember that your patients provide you with your living.

Confidentiality

Confidentiality is vital. The patient must be able to rely on the doctor's discretion. Unless there are compelling reasons for doing so, information must not be disclosed to any one else, including close relatives, without the patient's permission. Generally accepted reasons for breaking confidence are:

(1) telling close relatives about a serious diagnosis like cancer, when it may be necessary to plan care;
(2) where the rights of the community override those of the individual—e.g., the epileptic who insists on driving a lorry.

Everybody has the right to confidentiality—even children.

Willingness to give a good service

A good service, willingly given, does wonders for the doctor–patient relationship. The patient who regards you as well-intentioned is more likely to accept your opinions about what is, or is not necessary in the way of treatment or visits.

Sensitivity

To function well as a personal doctor you have to make a conscious effort to understand your patients' feelings and the way they think.

Dealing with symptoms at a superficial level can make life easier, but you are likely to miss the real reasons for the consultation and impair your ability to treat the whole person.

- Give more time for listening rather than talking.
- Open questions allow patients more scope for expressing themselves—for instance, 'What do you feel?' gives the patient more scope than 'Do you feel tense?'

Honesty

In any healthy relationship both parties should be as honest as possible with each other. Very often it is the doctor's emotions that prevent an honest exchange and communications may break down. Patients may feel isolated and rejected if they think that the truth is being withheld.

The skill in handling this lies in being able to determine what the patient really wants to know. A non-specific question like 'What do you know about your illness?' gives the patient an opportunity to ask for more information. In general, specific questions from the patients should be given honest replies.

Responsibility

It is your professional duty to help your patients appropriately and to the best of your ability. This does not mean that you have to respond to frivolous requests for housing transfers, but it does mean that you may have to spend time and energy trying to solve real problems. Referral to a consultant does not mean relinquishing responsibility. If advice or management seems to you be wrong then you must say so and take any appropriate action.

Sometimes relatives or other professionals may urge you to take courses of action which may not be in the best interests of your patient—e.g., getting a senile lady into hospital. If you think that it is kinder to keep her at home then you should do so—the patient's interests are paramount.

GP Colleagues

Partners

A practice cannot function properly if the partners are at logger-heads.

(1) Partners must be carefully chosen to be compatible.
(2) A good contract is essential.
(3) Work and income must be shared equitably.
(4) Decision-making must be democratic.
(5) Regular meetings should be held.
(6) Basic clinical and administrative policies are agreed and respected by all partners.

Neighbouring practices

Friction with neighbouring colleagues is much less likely if you get to know them socially and professionally.

Do not see patients of your colleagues, except in an emergency, without permission. This should also apply to private patients.

If you are in an out-of-hours rota make sure that you find out how the others like to have their patients managed. Never make overt or implied criticisms of your colleagues' treatment. Patients are skilful at playing one doctor off against another. Careful notes must be kept and given to the patient's doctor.

Private Practice

Regulations

(1) You cannot charge your NHS patients for any medical service even if in your view it is outside the normal range of services.
(2) You can charge for private certificates, private prescriptions and medical examinations for employment and driving.
(3) Some GPs remove a patient temporarily from their list so that they can provide a service, like vasectomy, for a fee.

Ethics

Remember that the patients who do come to see you privately are probably on someone else's NHS list and it is wise to get their permission and to find out about any current treatment.

Private clinics and abortion services

Pregnancy counselling clinics now exist in every large city. Some are run by charities but many are commercial. They will usually see patients without a referral letter and their interpretation of the abortion law is liberal.

After the initial interview the patient is normally sent to an associate private clinic that is licensed for abortion.

Family Planning Clinics

Organisation

Family planning clinics were originally run by a charity, but are now financed by the district health authority. Patients may attend without a referral letter, but most clinics are careful to inform the GP about any treatment.

If the GP is asked if there are any contra-indications to using the pill, it is then the GP's legal responsibility to check up on this and to reply if necessary.

Fringe Medicine

Ethics

Medical practitioners are not allowed to enter into any formal relationship with non-registered practitioners.

If you think that a patient may benefit from manipulation or acupuncture it is best to refer to a practitioner who is also medically qualified. If one is not available then allow the patient to choose whom to consult.

Do not be afraid to recommend unconventional treatment if you think that it is appropriate. Nevertheless, you must be alert to the fact that your patient may be exploited or may be subjected to treatment that may be dangerous.

The Registrar of Births and Deaths

Part of the registrar's job is to monitor the issuing of death certificates and he cannot register a death if the certificate is unsatisfactory in any way.

Certification procedure

(1) Avoid delay in issuing the certificate.

(2) Certificate is usually taken to the registrar by relatives, but it is the doctor's responsibility to make sure that it gets there.
(3) Use legible handwriting.
(4) Make sure the diagnosis is compatible with the international classification of diseases.
(5) Do not issue a certificate if you have any suspicions that the death was not natural.

The Coroner

Normally you should communicate with the coroner through the coroner's officer. The easiest way to establish contact is to telephone the local police station.

Reasons for reporting deaths

(1) Sudden, unexplained or unexpected deaths or where the doctor has not attended within 14 days.
(2) Unnatural abortions.
(3) Where accidents or injuries have contributed to death.
(4) Where there were industrial diseases or war pensioners' injuries.
(5) Deaths after anaesthetic or operation.
(6) Where there were drug mishaps or abuse, alcoholism or poisoning.
(7) Where persons were in legal custody.
(8) Stillbirth after 24 weeks.
(9) Where there is any suspicion of crime or suicide.

When in doubt, report. Very often the coroner will authorise you to issue a certificate if you think that the cause of death was natural.

Insurance Companies

Once a patient has authorised the insurance company to obtain a report you must provide an honest account of the facts. It would be reasonable, however, to point out to your patient any serious problems before you complete the report.

Reports

All the notes must be carefully perused so that an accurate summary of the medical history can be made.

Use the opportunity to put a summary in the record envelope and to get the contents in order.

Examinations

A full examination takes about 20 minutes. Book these at the end of surgery or at a separate session.

The practice nurse can do height, weight and urine tests.

Industry

The type and conditions of work can affect the health of your patients in many ways. Make an effort to look around local factories so that you get to know more about working conditions.

Improve patient care by:

(1) making a note of the patients' occupations on the records;
(2) asking about hazards at work;
(3) giving advice about minimising risks—for example, how to lift if there is any back trouble; and
(4) contact the factory doctor if working conditions need to be modified.

Most factory doctors are helpful and they can often arrange for routine treatments like injections or physiotherapy to be given at work. In smaller factories the doctors are often general practitioners who do one or two sessions of industrial work a week.

Social Services

Social services are financed and administered by the local authorities and they are quite separate from the health services.

Principal responsibilities are as set out below.

Children

Supervising the care of children in the community. Identifying those at risk. Taking them into care if necessary. Supervising fostering and adoption.

Elderly

The community care of the elderly. Providing home helps, wardens and old people's homes (*see* Part III: Accommodation).

Handicapped

The care of the physically or mentally handicapped (including mental subnormality). Providing aids such as walking frames, home helps, and house adaptations and sheltered workshops.

Mentally ill

Providing community care and hostels. Making applications for compulsory admissions.

Families

Care of families in financial, social or emotional trouble. Giving advice, counselling and welfare rights information.

Good GP/social worker cooperation depends on adequate communication. Have regular meetings and make sure that social workers have access to you when necessary. Understanding each other's responsibilities, abilities and limitations will make referrals more effective and relevant.

Schools

Ill children

Children with infectious diseases must be excluded from school. Home tuition may be available for long illnesses.
   If treatment is needed at school, contact the headmaster.

Teachers

Teachers are in contact with children all day and they can often provide good assessments of physical and emotional states. In problem cases a talk with the teacher can often produce much useful information.

Welfare officers

Many secondary schools now have welfare officers who undertake social worker type case work. They may also function as school attendance officers.

Counsellors

At least one teacher will have special training in counselling techniques—a good contact for emotional problems.

Child Guidance Clinics

Organisation

Originally run by the local authorities, the clinics are usually situated outside the hospital system. They deal with emotional problems in children under the age of 14 years.

Referrals may be made by GPs or directly by the education authorities.

Most clinics are orientated towards family therapy done by a team of social workers, pyschologists and child psychiatrists.

Voluntary Services

Services available include the following.

Samaritans. An emergency contact for emotionally upset patients.
Citizens Advice Bureaux. Give advice about legal and welfare rights problems.
Grapevine. Counselling for young people.
Old People's Welfare. Arrange clubs, outings, meals and social activities for the elderly.

The local council offices should be able to provide you with a complete list of voluntary organisations in your area.

7. PROFESSIONAL ORGANISATIONS

The General Medical Council

Set up in 1858, the General Medical Council (GMC) is a statutory body responsible directly to the Privy Council. Its chief function is to keep the Medical Register and its other roles stem from this. All medical practitioners have to be registered with the GMC. They pay an annual retention fee—£15 (1982).

The Medical Register is for full, limited or provisional registration (*see* pp. 34.)
Education. The GMC sets standards for education and undertakes the general surveillance of exams.
Overseas Doctors. The GMC ensures that overseas qualifications are commensurate with those in the UK.
Professional Conduct. There are no set rules but case law has been developed about what constitutes 'serious professional misconduct'. About 1000 complaints against doctors are made each year of which about 30–40 reach public hearings.
Types of Serious Professional Misconduct in order of frequency are as follows.

   (1) Abuse of alcohol or drugs.
   (2) Theft, fraud or dishonesty.
   (3) Disregard of care of patients.
   (4) Canvassing and advertising.
   (5) Improper relationships with patients (sexual or otherwise).
   (6) Indecency.

Sick Doctors. A new health committee is now able to deal with sick doctors without them having to appear in public.

British Medical Association

About 60% of the medical profession are members of the British Medical Association (BMA) and it is the principal medicopolitical body. The BMA:

(1) Negotiates with the government on pay and conditions of work in the NHS;
(2) Provides advice and guidance on many general and personal professional matters;
(3) Publishes the *British Medical Journal* (*BMJ*) and other journals and books;
(4) Organises national and local medicopolitical activities;
(5) Provides membership of most important governmental and professional committees.

Royal College of General Practitioners

The Royal College of General Practitioners (RCGP) is the academic voice and image of general practice. Founded in 1952, more than a quarter of GPs are now members or fellows.

(1) The MRCGP examination is held twice a year. There are written and oral parts. The pass rate is 60–70%.
(2) The RCGP publishes the college journal and numerous reports.
(3) The RCGP organises some research and also give advice to individuals undertaking research.
(4) Activities are organised locally at faculty level or centrally.
(5) RCGP is concerned with the supervision of vocational training through the JCPT.

General Medical Services Committee

The General Medical Services Committee (GMSC) is really a sub-committee of the BMA, but is organised to represent all GPs–members and non-members. It negotiates for general practitioners with the government about pay and conditions of work.

Local Medical Committee

The Local Medical Committee (LMC) is elected by all local general practitioners to represent their views to the FPC and other NHS bodies. It has representatives on the FPC.

The annual conference of LMCs shapes national policy about general practice matters. This is implemented through the GMSC.

Family Practitioner Committee

The Family Practitioner Committee (FPC) is the statutory body of the NHS that administers general practice and contracts with GPs to provide services. It pays GPs, arranges pensions and reimburses for staff, rent and rates; supplies records, prescription pads, other forms and syringes; and receives and investigates complaints from patients. It also administers services provided by dentists, pharmacists and opticians.

Postgraduate Medical Centres

Postgraduate medical centres are based on local district general hospitals. They are administered by the clinical tutor who is appointed by the university, through the postgraduate committee.

The BMA and the RCGP

Both have local organisations, but activities depend on local enthusiasm, which varies considerably.

8. THE LAW, CONFIDENTIALITY, CONSENT AND COMPLAINTS

The Law

Registration with the General Medical Council

All medical practitioners have to be recognised as such and registered with the General Medical Council (GMC).

Forms of registration

Provisional Registration. For doctors before completing their preregistration year.
Full Registration. After satisfactory completion of the preregistration year, or the equivalent for overseas doctors.
Limited Registration. For overseas doctors with recognised qualifications. It is limited in time and place, to certain hospital appointments and to specialty. Limited registration does not allow work in general practice.

Defence organisations

Although not compulsory in law it is essential that any doctor in practice or a trainee is a member of a defence organisation (Medical Defence Union, Medical Protection Society, Medical and Dental Defence Union of Scotland). Defence organisations provide:

(1) Medicolegal advice and support.
(2) Legal representation at courts and inquiries.
(3) Financial indemnity for professional claims.

Drugs and prescribing

Registration with the GMC allows privileges of possessing and prescribing drugs which are coupled with certain rules and codes.

NHS General Practice

- Prescribing is a statutory part of the GP's services.
- There is an obligation to prescribe any necessary drugs. The GP has the privilege of deciding what is necessary. This can be challenged by the patient.
- Patients are expected to provided medicines that could be regarded as 'household remedies' for themselves.
- Borderline substances are preparations like shampoos which can be prescribed only for certain conditions.

Controlled drugs

Make sure you are familiar with the provisions of the Dangerous Drugs and the Misuse of Drugs Acts.
Scheduled Drugs. The following must be adhered to.

(1) Register must be kept of all drugs you obtain.
(2) All the prescriptions must be handwritten by the prescriber with the strength and the total amount to be dispensed written in letters and figures.
(3) Must be kept in a locked receptacle.

Addicts

It is an offence to prescribe scheduled drugs to a known addict.

Addicts must be notified to the chief medical officer at the Home Office within seven days.

Beware of strangers with plausible stories asking for prescriptions for controlled drugs.

General

Never prescribe for yourself and take extra care when prescribing for family or friends. Make sure that they are not being treated by another general practitioner.

Confidentiality

Confidentiality is fundamental to the doctor/patient relationship. Doctors who break confidentiality could be sued in court or reported to the GMC. The following are some aspects of ethical conduct.

- Beware of loose talk about patients within the practice team or among family and friends.
- Do not give information to anybody, including relatives, without the patient's permission, unless it is necessitated by the circumstances of an acute or grave illness.
- Get written permission to supply reports to insurance companies, solicitors and even courts, unless subpoenaed by the court.
- Take care when reporting to employers. Whenever possible send your report to another doctor.
- In certain circumstances the safety of the community may override the individual's right to confidentiality.

Consent

In general a patient must give informed consent before any investigation or therapeutic procedure may be carried out.

- Up to the age of 16, parents are responsible for the wellbeing of their children and it is for them to give consent for treatment and investigations. There may be an ethical dilemma when this conflicts with the child's right to confidentiality. The merits of the case must then dictate the correct course of action, the child's interests being paramount.

- Informed consent implies that patients have a clear understanding about what is being done to and for them.
- In an emergency any necessary measures may be carried out.
- Take particular care to obtain consent for:

  (1) involvement in research—including drug trials;
  (2) the provision of medical reports;
  (3) post mortem examinations; and
  (4) the use of organs for transplants.

Complaints

Complaints against a GP may be made in the following ways

To the practice where they are usually dealt with, informally.
To the Family Practitioner Committee where they may be dealt with informally by the chairman or may be referred for a formal hearing by the Medical Services Committee.
To the General Medical Council in the case of alleged serious professional misconduct.
To the Courts where a civil action may ensue.

In all cases the advice of a professional defence organisation should be sought.

Therapeutic abortion

The role of the GP is to act as a counsellor and then to make a referral to an NHS hospital or to a private clinic if a termination of pregnancy is indicated. If you have a conscientious objection to abortion it is reasonable to offer the patient the opportunity of a consultation with another doctor.

The Abortion Act (1968)

Two medical practitioners have to certify (on form HSA1) that a termination is necessary for one of the following reasons.

(1) That continuing the pregnancy involves a risk to life or of physical or mental injury greater than if the pregnancy were terminated.
(2) That continuing the pregnancy involves a risk of mental or

37

physical injury to existing children greater than if the pregnancy were terminated.

(3) That there is a substantial risk that the child may be born with a serious mental or physical handicap.

Practical points

(1) In some areas terminations are difficult to obtain under the NHS. The response and medical standards are more predictable in the private sector.

(2) The earlier the termination is done the lower the likelihood of complications.

(3) No consent is required from the parents. In a girl under the age of 16 termination may still be carried out in spite of parental opposition—but get advice from your defence organisation.

PART II
INVESTIGATION AND MANAGEMENT

9. ACCESS TO HOSPITAL LABORATORY AND RADIOLOGY FACILITIES

Differences From Hospital Practice

Differences may arise for the following reasons:

(1) Many illnesses seen by the GP are minor and self-limiting, thus investigation may be of no value in guiding treatment and the patient may well have recovered before the results become available.

(2) Many GPs are some distance from the nearest hospital. Special arrangements must therefore be made to transport specimens to the laboratory or the patient may have to travel to the department, which causes them expense and inconvenience.

(3) Much of all disease is seen only by the GP. The investigative services would soon be overloaded if GPs were not selective in their use.

(4) Nevertheless, selective and judicious use of open access to the hospital facilities enables the GP to investigate and manage many patients himself, thus increasing his own job satisfaction, reducing the load on outpatient departments, and saving patients both time and expense.

Ordering Investigations

When ordering investigations consider the following criteria:

(1) Is this investigation necessary to clinch an important diagnosis—e.g. suspected urinary tract infection in a small child?

(2) Is this investigation necessary in order to monitor control of a chronic disorder—e.g. blood glucose in a diabetic?

(3) Is this investigation necessary in order to exclude serious disease—e.g. an ESR (erythrocyte sedimentation rate) in suspected temporal arteritis, a chest x-ray examination to exclude a carcinoma of the lung?

(4) Will the results of this investigation lead to a change in treatment?—e.g. trichomonas in a high vaginal swab?

(5) Will the inconvenience to the patient and the cost of the

41

procedure be justified in relation to the value of the results obtained—e.g. barium meal in vague dyspepsia?

(6) Are there any special features of the investigation which require the patient to be provided with prior detailed instructions?—e.g. overnight fasting before lipoprotein estimation? (If in doubt, look it up or telephone the department for advice.)

(7) Can the specimen be delivered to the laboratory at a suitable time for them to process it—e.g. reliable estimations of serum potassium cannot be performed on an old specimen of blood?

Bacteriology

The use of a transport medium improves the chances of successful culture. Specimens taken after the patient has started on antibiotics are most unlikely to yield positive results.

Throat swabs are not routinely indicated because up to 75% will fail to demonstrate a streptococcus. The decision to prescribe penicillin (or erythromycin) should be made on clinical grounds (degree of pain, systemic upset, cervical lymphadenopathy). If the pharyngitis is exceptionally severe or persistent than a swab may be indicated, but a full blood count and Monospot or Paul-Bunnell tests are more relevant investigations.

Ear swabs are indicated only if there is a chronic discharge from the ear. Acute otitis media is best treated by amoxycillin if the patient is under 2-years-old, when *Haemophilus influenzae* is a more likely pathogen, or penicillin thereafter.

Eye swabs are not normally required in general practice because chloramphenicol eye drops or ointment eradicate most likely pathogens. However, beware gonococcal infection or chlamydia in small babies with sticky eyes.

Sputum culture is rarely helpful and may be confusing. Nevertheless, if the patient fails to respond to the antibiotic prescribed then culture may be indicated. If tuberculosis needs to be excluded then a series of cultures for acid-fast bacilli are required. One specimen is not enough.

Mid-stream urine (MSU) specimens are essential in order to prove urinary tract infection. Even so, 50% of adult women with symptoms of dysuria and frequency will not demonstrate significant bacteriuria. As with sore throats, it is usual to treat on clinical grounds (degree of discomfort, systemic upset, etc.) with trimethoprim, co-trimoxazole or amoxycillin, without waiting for the results of culture. The most reliable method is to use a dip-slide or dip-spoon technique to overcome the problem of contamination which may be aggravated by delay in reaching the laboratory.

Remember that asymptomatic bacteria is important only in children and pregnant women, otherwise treatment is directed towards relief of symptoms and repeated MSUs are not usually indicated in the absence of symptoms.

Stool culture is required only:

(1) on public health grounds if the patient is a food handler;
(2) on epidemiological grounds, e.g. an outbreak of food poisoning;
(3) if the patient has recently returned from the tropics;
(4) if the diarrhoea is severe and persistent.

Remember to ask for stool microscopy for ova and parasites as well as bacteriological culture.

Skin swabs are rarely indicated because the treatment of boils and impetigo will not be influenced by the swab results. Flucloxacillin or erythromycin are most effective against staphylococci, while tetracycline ointment is the local preparation of choice.

Leg ulcer may grow a variety of opportunistic organisms. Treatment of the ulcer on general principles of support and pressure bandaging is most important. If a pure culture of a pathogenic organism is isolated then systemic antibiotics are preferable to local sprays and ointments, because local applications are especially prone to cause skin sensitivity reactions in these circumstances.

High vaginal swabs may be useful in pelvic inflammatory disease and, especially, in vulvovaginitis. Monilia is frequently isolated but trichomonas organisms tend to die en route to the laboratory and are best demonstrated under a microscope at the surgery. It has recently been shown that the only other important pathogen causing vaginitis is *Gardnerella vaginalis*, a facultative anaerobe. Monilia is best treated by local treatment with nystatin or clotrimazole and trichomonas and gardnerella both respond well to oral metronidazole.

Cervical and urethral swabs should be taken, preferably on a charcoal swab and dispatched rapidly to the laboratory in a transport medium if the gonococcus is to be isolated. It must be emphasised, however, that satisfactory exclusion of gonorrhoea in the face of clinical suspicion requires attendance at a medical genitourinary clinic and the patient must be advised accordingly.

Malaria parasites can be demonstrated in blood collected in an ordinary EDTA bottle and transferred promptly to the laboratory. Try to collect the specimen as the fever is rising. Treatment of acute malaria in general practice is usually easy and rapid with chloroquin, but beware of falciparum infection if the patient comes from East or West Africa, South-East Asia or South America. The laboratory will usually also test for G-6-PD deficiency since the eradication of benign tertian malaria due to *Plasmodium vivax*, *ovale* or *malariae* requires a course of primaquine, a drug which can cause haemolysis in patients who are deficient in the enzyme.

Virus culture is normally required only for research purposes and needs special collection and transport methods. Consult your local laboratory for information.

Serology

Rising titres on paired sera may be required occasionally to confirm specific viral infections, notably rubella in early pregnancy (see pp. 143–4). Patients with vague symptoms and recurrent pyrexia may be investigated in this way to exclude brucellosis, toxoplasmosis or the milder enteric fevers, while an occasional anti-streptolysin O titre is still needed in the investigation of suspected rheumatic fever.

Infectious mononucleosis may be diagnosed on clinical grounds, together with abnormal monocytes on a blood film. However, it is usual to confirm the diagnosis by requesting a Paul-Bunnell or Monospot test for heterophil antibodies in the second week of the illness.

Testing for auto-immune antibodies may be required specifically in connective tissue disorders such as rheumatoid arthritis (RA latex, Rose-Waaler, ANF), in hepatitis (Australia antigen), and in endocrine disease (thyroid antibodies).

Serological tests for syphilis are rarely performed in general practice today except as part of routine antenatal care. It is important to realise that Wasserman or Kahn tests may produce biological false–positive results in various immunological disorders. Venereal Disease Research Laboratory. (VDRL) and Treponemal immobilisation tests (TIT) are more specific.

HLA-B27 tissue type is a common finding in association with some infrequent rheumatological disorders, especially ankylosing spondylitis.

Immunological pregnancy testing may be performed either in the practice or at the local laboratory, but it is only clinically necessary where the diagnosis of pregnancy must be made as quickly as possible, e.g. if termination is to be considered, or if there may be a problem such as possible ectopic pregnancy or miscarriage.

Haematology

Use the appropriate form and specimen bottles supplied by your laboratory. Transfer the specimen as soon as possible because blood cells degenerate quickly.

Remember to request platelet counts specifically if required, since they are not performed routinely. ESRs may be more easily and accurately measured at the surgery.

Pay particular attention to the haematologist's comments and consult him if in doubt about further investigations.

Anaemia is common and often asymptomatic. It has been estimated that only one case in four will be known to the GP. Women in the productive years and the elderly are the two most vulnerable groups, but premature infants, post-gastrectomy patients and those with chronic illnesses, poor diet and chronic blood loss are also at risk. Of cases in general practice 91% are due to iron deficiency, 7% to megaloblastic anaemia and 2% to the rarer haemolytic anaemias. Management includes accurate diagnosis of any underlying lesion and, in addition, further haematological investigations such as serum iron and iron-binding capacity or serum B_{12} and folic acid may be required. All patients should be followed-up at regular intervals.

Leucocyte counts may be useful in confirming infection, distinguishing between infections, monitoring chemotherapy and excluding leukaemia in rare instances.

Eosinophilia may be indicative of allergy or parasitic infestation.

Anticoagulant control is easily managed in general practice provided that communication between the laboratory and the practice is good.

Cytology

Cervical smears are frequently performed by the GP. All women over 35, and those who have had more than three pregnancies, are encouraged to attend every 5 years, the doctor being paid a fee for each examination. Otherwise, smears are usually performed in the course of routine contraceptive and maternity care and as part of a gynaecological examination. The cervix must be clearly visualised, the spatula must be rotated through the full 360° in the cervical os, and the specimen must be fixed and dried before transport to the laboratory.

Sputum and urine specimens may be submitted for cytological investigation if malignancy is suspected.

Material obtained from minor surgical procedures should be submitted for histology.

Biochemistry

Biochemical tests have become more important to GPs in recent years. Many laboratories now report several results on each specimen of blood submitted because of the widespread use of the auto-analyser.

Urea and electrolyte estimations are most commonly required in patients with renal or cardiac conditions, especially if they are maintained on diuretic therapy. It is recommended that serum potassium should be monitored every 3–6 months in these patients, especially if they are also taking digoxin or are not on potassium supplements.

Serum calcium specimens should be taken without a tourniquet—otherwise false results may be obtained. The most common indication in general practice is when renal calculi are found, but another important area is in terminal care. Hypercalcaemia due to multiple bone secondaries may cause nausea and vomiting and can be effectively treated by administering a steroid.

Enzyme estimations are increased by haemolysis. They are most commonly used in investigating cardiac and hepatic disease.

Lipoprotein profiles require overnight fasting. Marked abnormalities, as in familial hyperlipoproteinaemias, are significant risk factors for arteriopathy.

Serum creatinine is a better simple guide to renal function than blood urea.

Blood glucose estimation. Fasting or two hours post-prandial is required for the diagnosis of diabetes. Do *not* rely on urine testing only. Regular self-monitoring using electronic meters is gradually superseding urine testing in established diabetics, especially if they are pregnant or their condition is unstable.

Serum acid phosphatase is raised in metastatic bone disease from carcinoma of the prostate. It should be specifically requested because it is not usually done routinely.

Serum gamma-glutamyl transpeptidase is a useful simple screening test for excessive alcohol intake, taken in conjunction with an otherwise unexplained macrocytosis on the blood film.

Modern thyroid function tests including T4, T3 uptake and the free thyroxine index are much more reliable than older methods such as basal metabolic rate (BMR) and protein-bound iodine (PBI). Thyroid-stimulating hormone (TSH) estimation is now possible on very small amounts of blood and is available for screening neonates. It is likely that more cases of mild hyperthyroidism, and especially hypothyroidism in the elderly, will be detected and treated because of the widespread availability of these tests. Monitoring of treated hypothyroidism requires regular TSH measurements at six-monthly intervals.

Radiology

Avoid unnecessary radiation. It is often possible to review the patient a few days after a traumatic episode and thus avoid radiography.

Remember the 10-day rule for women of child-bearing age. It is your responsibility to state the last menstrual period (LMP) on the request form.

State relevant clinical findings and reason for request on form.

Mark the request form *URGENT* only if clinically indicated, not just for social convenience.

Treat an x-ray request as a consultation with a consultant radiologist, *not* as an order to a technician. He or she will advise you if special views are required, if an ultrasonic scan would be more helpful in the particular circumstances, or if an alternative investigation should be performed first—e.g. sigmoidoscopy before a barium enema.

Negative findings may be important in order to reassure both the

47

patient and the doctor. Nevertheless, there are cheaper and safer placebos available.

Plain x-rays do not require prior preparation. Remember that negative findings on x-ray films of bones and joints do not exclude disease—e.g. 40% of a vertebra may need to be invaded by metastases before it is radiologically demonstrable; x-ray films of the lumbar spine in acute backache or sciatica will show only long-established changes; brain damage can occur in the absence of a skull fracture.

Barium swallows and meals do not give infallible results. Endoscopic examination may be preferable if it is readily available. Gastric ulcers must be followed up radiologically or endoscopically, but duodenal ulcers may be safely monitored by response to treatment.

Oral cholecystography is contraindicated if the patient is jaundiced. Many radiologists now consider ultrasound to be a preferable initial investigation.

Intravenous urography is likely to be unsatisfactory if renal function is impaired. The radiologist must be informed accordingly so that a larger dose of contrast medium can be used.

Mammography may be helpful in some clinically benign or doubtful breast lumps, or as a screening technique in patients with a high risk of breast cancer. It is most reliable in post-menopausal women.

Ultrasound investigation is now widely used in obstetrics for estimating the stage of gestation, demonstrating the placental site, excluding multiple pregnancy and some fetal abnormalities and establishing viability after a threatened miscarriage.

10. INVESTIGATIONS WITHIN THE PRACTICE

Investigations in the surgery may be used to look for diseases which are best treated at a presymptomatic stage (screening), or for diagnosing and monitoring established disease. Some will be undertaken by a nurse or health visitor and some by a doctor or by all these working together.

Screening of Apparently Healthy People

There are few conditions where it is worthwhile to screen whole unselected populations. There is no point in screening for a condition which, even if common, is not amenable to treatment—such as carcinoma of the lung. Rare conditions are worth screening for only if presymptomatic treatment is of proved value. Phenylketonuria comes into this category. A routine medical examination of an asymptomatic adult is useful only to detect hypertension. If he is obese or smokes, these facts will already be known to him. As yet there is no evidence that screening for carcinoma of the breast is worthwhile. Whatever the facts, screening for carcinoma of the cervix has now become standard practice. Screening of selected individuals for selected conditions is clearly useful, and general practice the ideal setting from which to carry it out (see Table 10.1).

- Within any 3 year period 90% of people see their general practitioner so, if they take advantage of the opportunities, the vast majority of patients will be screened within a short period without special appointments.
- An alternative method is to set up a screening programme.
- A computer may be used in conjunction with either system.

Diagnosis and Treatment of Disease

Height and weight

Standard scales and a ruler fixed to a wall are essential in any surgery. It is useful to have them marked both in metric and imperial units. Charts of the normal range and percentile charts are useful, especially when reassuring parents, anxious about a lean child, who may well be on the 50 percentile line and making steady progress.

Vision

Snellen's types for distant vision, near vision and Ishihara for testing colour vision can all be used by the practice nurse. Care is necessary to ensure that the distance is correct and one eye covered in using the lists for distant and near vision.

Audiometry

An audiometer is easy to use in adults and in children over 6 years,

Table 10.1 *Screening*

Condition	Test	Age/interval	Where usually carried out	By whom
CHILDREN				
Phenylketonuria	Guthrie	6-days-old	Hospital maternity ward	Midwife
Congenital hypothyroidism	Serum TSH	6-days-old	Hospital maternity ward	Midwife
Congenital physical abnormality (e.g. dislocated hip)	Physical examination	1. Birth	Hospital maternity department	Obstetric or paediatric HO or GP
		2. 10-days-old	Home	GP
		3. 6-weeks-old	Well baby clinic	GP
		4. 6-months-old	Well baby clinic	GP
Deafness/visual problems	Hearing test/ visual acuity	1. 8-months-old	Well baby clinic	Health visitor
		2. 4-years-old	Well baby clinic	Health visitor
		3. 7-years-old	Well baby clinic or school	Health visitor or school nurse
ADULTS				
Hypertension	Blood pressure	Every five years	Surgery or occupational health clinic	GP or nurse MO or nurse
Carcinoma of the cervix	Cervical smear	Every five years from age 20 to 35 then every three years	Surgery	GP or nurse

old although time and patience are required. Younger children are often difficult to test.

Blood pressure

Mercury and aneroid sphygmomanometers are equally efficient but both types need checking from time to time. There seems little point in using a random zero sphygmomanometer except for research purposes. Nurses are perfectly capable of taking blood pressure measurements but everyone in the practice should make sure he or she is using the same end points. It is important to use a small cuff for measuring blood pressure in children.

Respiratory function

Peak flow meter. This is a simple gadget that gives a reasonably reliable measurement of peak expiratory flow rate measured in litres per minute. It is a useful objective guide to the success of treatment in individual patients with asthma. It can be used to frighten smokers, if a chart of normals for height and age is kept. From time to time, certain drug companies make peak flow meters available to general practitioners free of charge.

Electrocardiography

This is invaluable in the diagnosis of arrythmias and of chest pain, although its limitations must be borne in mind (a normal ECG does not rule out a diagnosis of angina and typical changes following infarction may be delayed). Nurses with special training are efficient at making ECG recordings. Interpretation is done by the doctor. It is usually possible to send difficult tracings to a consultant cardiologist for a report.

Urine testing

Dip sticks have made urine testing a simple matter, but certain precautions must be taken if the results are to be reliable. The sample should be a 'clean catch' one, if possible, and must be passed into a clean container. Albustix must be read immediately and Clinistix must be fresh. Once opened they deteriorate quickly and can give a false–negative result. Clinistix are not suitable for quantitative testing. Acetone in urine can be detected by Acetest tablets, if they are dry and in good condition. Bile can be detected by shaking the urine and looking for yellow froth or by using Ictotest tablets.

Culture and microscopy. There is no reason why these should not be carried out in the surgery and the results may be more reliable than when samples are delayed by being sent to the hospital laboratory. Most doctors find it easier to use the hospital laboratory facilities, however, and few now do their own culture and microscopy.

Vaginal swabs

A high vaginal swab, transferred to a slide and examined under a microscope immediately may show trichomonas, which might have died by the time the swab reached the laboratory. The gonococcus is more difficult to identify and if venereal disease is possible, the patient should be advised to attend a special clinic.

Blood sugar estimation

Blood sugar may be estimated with reasonable accuracy using sticks with a colour chart or electronic comparing device. The sticks must be fresh and the timing and other instructions followed with scrupulous care.

11. PRINCIPLES OF TREATMENT

Most patients seen by general practitioners do not need prescribed medication, either for the relief of symptoms or to treat disease. Nevertheless, if a patient is anxious or distressed the doctor may feel the need to give a prescription as a token of his sympathy and his willingness to help. He may believe that this is what the patient expects. He may feel that he lacks the necessary time for the detailed explanation that would be needed if he were not to provide a prescription.

Those patients who do need medication usually have to be left in sole charge of administering it. Its efficacy may depend on their appreciation of its importance combined with intelligent and conscientous interpretation of the doctor's instructions.

It is therefore much more difficult in general practice than in hospital to use drugs in a completely logical way and special care is needed to ensure safe and sensible prescribing and administration.

It may be helpful to work out a personal code of practice for prescribing. Something basic and simple, along the lines of the list below, would do to start with. More detail can then be added if necessary.

(1) Prescribe nothing unless there is a clear clinical indication for it—i.e. an expectation that it will materially alter the course of the illness or relieve suffering.

(2) Choose the cheapest satisfactory form of the drug available.

(3) If the clinical indication is for a placebo, make sure that it is both safe and cheap.

(4) Make sure the patient agrees to take the drug, understands what it is for, and how it should be taken.

The doctor needs to bear in mind what a patient needs to know about any drug.

- How should the drug be given?—i.e. by what route, how often, when, in relation to meals, for how long? Is it a short course or should it be continued indefinitely?
- What effect is it likely to have on the illness?—i.e. immediate cure, delayed cure, relief of symptoms (complete or partial), no obvious effect?
- Should the drug be continued after the condition appears to have resolved?
- If the drug is to be taken 'as required', exactly what is the indication for a dose? How often may it be repeated? What is the maximum total dose in 24 hours?
- What side effects are to be expected, are likely, are possible but nothing to worry about, should be reported to the doctor, should make me stop taking the drug?
- How important is it to take the drug? What will happen if it is not taken?

To practise efficient prescribing, the doctor needs to have a clear idea of the following:

- Why exactly has the patient come to see the doctor?
  Is it because he is anxious about the meaning of a symptom (e.g. whether the headache is due to a brain tumour)?

Is he simply seeking symptomatic relief?
Does he want to discuss some other problem?
- What is the diagnosis?
  Is medication likely to be useless, helpful, important, essential?
- If infection is present
  what is the most likely organism?
  what is it likely to be sensitive to?
  would the patient recover without a drug?
- If medication is not indicated, does the patient understand why?
  What can he do for himself?
- If medication is important, e.g. in hypertension,
  does the patient share the doctor's enthusiasm and agree to take the drug?
  Is he capable of remembering to take it regularly?
- If the timing of doses is important and individually variable, e.g. sodium cromoglycate in asthma, does the patient understand how the drug works and how to work out, for himself, when to take it?

This sounds time-consuming but it can be covered quite briefly and if the end-result is that people become better educated about drugs and the management of minor illness, fewer patients will attend the surgery for problems which they can deal with quite competently without the help of a doctor.

12. COMMON CLINICAL PROBLEMS

The new trainee in general practice often has considerable difficulty in reorientating his clinical approach and thinking from that acquired in hospital.

GPs are often apologetic because they do not have the time to follow the routine which they were taught as students—a detailed history and examination followed by appropriate investigations. A little reflection, however, will show that the approach of the orthopaedic surgeon, for instance, is very different from that of the gynaecologist, while the ophthalmologist and the thoracic surgeon have little in common. Each has had to modify his approach to clinical medicine in the light of his specialist functioin. The general practitioner is no exception.

The issue for the new entrant to general practice is, therefore, how to adopt his basic clinical approach in a way which is safe, effective and relevant for primary care. Statistically, we know that most conditions seen in primary care are minor and self-limiting, while many of the others are chronic and persistent. Major life-threatening conditions are uncommon but it is essential that they should not be overlooked. Unfortunately, there is often little or no difference between the early symptoms of a major condition and the definitive symptoms of a minor condition. A cough, for example, may signify anything from a minor respiratory infection to a carcinoma of the bronchus.

In the section which follows we have chosen some common presenting symptoms and suggested a clinical approach that seems appropriate and relevant in the context of primary care. In the end every GP has to devise his or her own approach but these suggestions provide a starting point for consideration.

Emergencies are dealt with in Chapter 14.

Headache

There is a persistent myth, common among patients and even some doctors, that headache is a symptom of a raised blood pressure. With the exception of the rare case of malignant hypertension there is no basis for this belief.

Common causes

Tension with or without anxiety/depression. Usually described as a tight band or pressure on top of the head or pain and tenderness in the occipital region.

Migraine. A diagnostic point is the recurrent nature of the headache, occurring in bouts. The classical prodromal triad—unilateral headache, nausea and vomiting—is less common than partial syndromes.

Toxic. Caused by infections, drugs (remember overuse of ergotamine), and alcohol

Secondary to other conditions affecting the head and neck—e.g. sinusitis, cervical spondylosis, ocular conditions.

Less common causes

Temporal arteritis in the elderly.
Meningitis.
Raised intracranial pressure such as tumours, subdural haematoma, subarachnoid haemorrhage.

Pitfalls

- Pain due to raised intracranial pressure may not be severe initially. Persistent headache or pain which is unusual in type or frequency for that patient should arouse suspicion.
- Subarachnoid haemorrhage may present as severe migraine.
- Elderly patients with temporal arteritis may complain only of vague pains—remember the association with polymyalgia rheumatica.
- Children with space-occupying lesions may suffer remarkably mild headaches. Vomiting may be appreciable but the periodic syndrome is much more common than brain tumours.

Approach

History

Establish the site, frequency and intensity of headache, and ask about any associated symptoms, e.g. visual disturbance, vomiting, and any precipitating and relieving factors.

Examination

Examine the head, neck and fundi, and take the blood pressure (the patient expects this, and it provides an opportunity for screening).

Management

Manage as appropriate to the diagnosis. If you are not sure, there is no harm in waiting and reviewing the patient a few days later.

Pain In The Chest

This symptom causes considerable anxiety in patients, especially young or middle-aged men who are worried about heart disease.

Common causes

Musculoskeletal
> Trauma, muscular spasm due to anxiety.
> Viral myalgia (mild, Bornholm-type illness).
> Cough fractures (suspected secondaries).
> Tender costal cartilages (Tietze's syndrome).
> Referred pain, often girdle distribution, due to disorders of the thoracic spine.

Infective. More often discomfort or soreness rather than pain.
Herpes zoster

Less common causes

Cardiovascular. Ischaemic cardiac pain, pericarditis, pulmonary embolus.
Respiratory. Pleurisy, pneumonia, spontaneous pneumothorax.
Oesophageal reflux. Hiatus hernia.

Pitfalls

• In herpes zoster, quite severe pain may precede the rash by some days.
• Ischaemic cardiac pain is often described as 'indigestion'. If 'indigestion' is severe enough to wake the patient up or to persist all night it is much more likely to represent angina or myocardial infarction.
• Ischaemic cardiac pain may be felt in the back, shoulders, arms, neck or face instead of—or as well as—in the central chest area.
• Left-sided inframammary pain is much more likely to be due to anxiety than angina.

Approach

History

Establish the site, onset, character and duration of pain, and ask about any associated symptoms—nausea, vomiting, faintness—and any precipitating and relieving factors.

Examination (essential to relieve anxiety)

Examine the cardiovascular system (CVS), respiratory system (RS) and blood pressure (BP).

Investigation

ECG may be useful to demonstrate changes of infarction or arrhythmia, *but* remember a normal ECG at rest *does not exclude angina or early infarction*. It may help to reassure the patient.

Cardiac enzymes should be repeated daily if infarction is suspected.

Chest x-ray examination is indicated in smokers, immigrants, old patients, those with signs of pleurisy or pneumonia and persistent pain associated with cough.

Management

Determine patient's fears and reassure as appropriate, but if in doubt review the patient's condition within hours or days as required.

Severe chest pain demands powerful remedies, i.e. opiates by injection.

Decision about hospital admission must be made on clinical grounds.

Cough

Most patients, or their parents, are more annoyed than worried by a cough. The temptation for the doctor is to prescribe rather than try to make a diagnosis.

Common causes

Upper respiratory tract infection. This is by far the most common cause of coughing, especially in children.

Bronchial irritation. Smoking and, less commonly, dust and fumes are common causes of persistent cough.

Asthma. In many patients cough rather than wheeze is the predominant symptom, especially if it occurs on exercise or at night.

Chronic bronchitis. The most common cause of a persistent, productive cough—especially if the patient is a smoker.

Less common causes

Pneumonia.
Tuberculosis. In immigrants, alcoholics and elderly men.
Carcinoma of bronchus. In smokers, remember to have a chest x-ray if cough or physical signs persist after acute infection.
Foreign bodies such as inhaled peanuts in toddlers.
Whooping cough. In children, which is often modified by immunisation.

Pitfalls

- Remember to think of allergy if the patient complains of frequent or persistent coughs and colds.
- Always consider the possibility of reversible airways obstruction, especially in children and elderly bronchitics.
- Remember that large numbers of eosinophils in sputum will colour it yellow, so allergy rather than infection may be the underlying cause of 'purulent' sputum.

Approach

History

Find out about smoking habits, and establish duration, severity and persistence of cough; nature, consistency and colour of sputum. Find out if there is an association of chest pain or breathlessness.

Examination

Check general appearance, whether there is any weight loss or clubbing, and examine upper respiratory tract, including ears and chest.

Investigation

Chest x-ray examination in smokers, immigrants, older patients, pleurisy, pneumonia, whooping cough.
Peak-flow readings in asthma and bronchitis, before and after treatment.
Examine sputum for eosinophils; cytology and culture may be useful occasionally.

Management

As appropriate, stop **patient** from smoking (and include parents). Remember that oral **fluids and** a humid atmosphere help expectoration and soothe cough, **and** most cough medicines are valueless but harmless.

Avoid giving antibiotics in uncomplicated upper respiratory tract infection (URTI).

Asthma requires bronchodilators and occasionally steroids, preferably by inhalation, rather than antibiotics.

Indigestion

Indigestion is a vague term used both by patients and doctors. It usually implies pain or discomfort felt in the epigastrium or lower chest. It may or may not be associated with heartburn, flatulence, nausea or vomiting.

Common causes

Dietary indiscretion. Certain highly spiced foods, e.g. curry, salads, new bread or tomatoes, may cause indigestion in susceptible people.
Alcohol is a common cause of recurrent indigestion.
Smoking.
Excessive tea, coffee or mineral water.
Drugs especially aspirin.
'*Stress*', anxiety, depression.

Less common causes

Peptic ulcer typically causes recurrent bouts of dyspepsia over a 5–10-year period.
Hiatus hernia is often symptomless, but may give rise to dyspepsia if there is acid reflux into oesophagus.
Gallbladder disease is frequently symptomless, but may cause dyspepsia, jaundice and severe biliary colic.
Pancreatitis is more common in alcoholics and diabetics.
Carcinoma of oesophagus, stomach or pancreas are usually associated with dysphagia, anorexia, weight loss and malaise.

Pitfalls

- Avoid confusion with angina.
- Remember how common is alcohol abuse.
- Beware of the older patient who develops dyspepsia for the first time in his life—he may well have a malignancy.
- Remember to inquire about drug intake, especially self-medication.

Approach

History

Establish location and radiation of pain, aggravating and relieving factors, relationship to meals.

Find out response to self-medication—milk, antacids, and establish whether there are associated symptoms, especially melaena.

Examination

Check upper respiratory tract (URT), tongue, cervical lymph nodes, and examine abdomen—often nil specific to find.

Investigation

Barium meal may be indicated if symptoms persist or malignancy is a possibility.

Gastroscopy may be a preferable initial investigation, depending on local conditions.

Ultrasound is the quickest and cheapest way to demonstrate gallstones.

If melaena is suspected check occult blood in faeces.

If anaemia is suspected check haemoglobin count.

Management

Tell patient to avoid smoking, drinking, drugs, specific foods.

Suggest regular small meals and frequent and liberal doses of antacid.

Patient should avoid stooping, corsets, or horizontal position if reflux oesophagitis.

Give no specific ulcer treatment, e.g. cimetidine, without radiological or endoscopic proof.

Advise patient that most cases of non-specific dyspepsia settle with a few days.

Approach

Acute

The GP must make a decision not necessarily a diagnosis.
Any signs of peritoneal irritation or obstruction indicates hospital admission even if the diagnosis is obscure.

Advise the patient to avoid food, emetics or purgatives.

Non-acute

Detailed history and careful examination is essential, but often the only treatment necessary is advice, especially dietary.

Investigations are indicated if the pain is persistent, unusual in that particular patient or associated with changes in bowel habit, bleeding or abdominal masses.

Abdominal Pain

Patients with abdominal pain are most likely to be worried about appendicitis or 'ulcers'. Older patients may have anxieties about cancer—they may be right.

Common causes

In young children. Colic may cause severe spasmodic pain, often related to feeding problems or infection.
In older children. Children may be 'little belly-achers', have the periodic syndrome—possibly equivalent to migraine—with recurrent central abdominal pain with or without vomiting.
In young adults. Indigestion may be caused by stress, alcohol, nicotine, caffeine, irregular unsuitable meals. It may also be caused by irritable bowel syndrome or dysmenorrhoea.
In elderly patients. Constipation or diverticulitis may be causes.

Less common causes

In young children. Urinary tract infection or intussusception may be responsible.

In adults. Patients may have gall bladder colic, renal colic, peptic ulcer, colitis, Crohn's disease.

In young women. Ectopic pregnancy, salpingitis or ovarian cysts may be causes.

In the elderly. An old person may have acute or subacute obstruction or ischaemic bowel.

All ages. Appendicitis may be responsible.

Pitfalls

● Remember that as a GP you often see illness in its early stages. A careful examination may disclose nothing but a few hours later signs may be present. Be prepared to review the case if pain is persistent.

● Intussusception is often subacute rather than acute and may present in the same way as gastroenteritis.

● Appendicitis often presents atypically. It may follow gastroenteritis. Diagnosis is particularly difficult in children, pregnant women and the elderly.

● Ectopic pregnancy may occur without the typical menstrual history.

● Remember extraneous causes—e.g. diabetic crisis, shingles.

Breast Lumps and Tenderness

A lump in the breast inevitably raises fears of cancer in most women. To allay anxiety it is important for the doctor to make a positive statement about his findings and proposed management.

Common causes

Normal cyclical changes (worse if premenstrual). There is a wide range of variation between women, and between cycles in the same woman.

Mammary dysplasia (cystic mastitis, fibroadenosis) may give rise to tenderness, thickening and cyst formation, age 25–50 years.

Less common causes

Fibroadenoma. A firm, painless, mobile mass occurring predominantly in women under 30.
Carcinoma. The hallmark is attachment to the skin or underlying tissues.
Breast abscess is usually in the lactating breast.
Physiological mastitis (neonate, puberty).

Pitfalls

• Carcinoma may occur in a woman with pre-existing mammary dysplasia.

Approach

History

Taking a family history is important, especially mother and sisters. Check her parity and lactation, and establish variability with cycle.

Examination

Both breasts and axillae should be examined, and establish shape, size, texture (whether soft, hard, cystic, or irregular) of lump if present. Find areas of tenderness. Look for axillary nodes.

Investigation

Mammography if there are no definite physical signs, and in patients with previous breast cancer, strong family history, breast pain or very large breasts. It is most reliable in post-menopausal women.

Management

All isolated, persistent breast lumps must be regarded as malignant until proved otherwise. If mastitis is probable, review post-menstrually, but if sure there is no malignancy, reassure strongly. If in doubt, refer to a specialist.

Dysuria and Frequency

Dysuria and frequency are most common in young adult women but are of most significance in children and adult men.

Common causes

'Cystitis', which may or may not be associated with significant bacteriuria.
Urethritis. Non-specific urethritis (NSU) or gonorrhoea in men.

Less common causes

Pyelonephritis. Fever and loin pain are typical features, more frequent in pregnancy, diabetics or in association with calculi.
Tuberculosis of genitourinary tract in immigrants.
Bladder malignancy, which is often associated with haematuria.
Prostatomegaly, prostatitis, carcinoma of prostate.
Epididymo-orchitis.

Pitfalls

● Urinary symptoms may be presented in lieu of an underlying sexual problem.
● Urinary tract infection can occur without localising symptoms, especially in small children.
● Prolapse in older women and prostatic problems in older men are often responsible for recurrent infections.
● Hormone deficiency in perimenopausal and post-menopausal women may cause recurrent urethral symptoms.

Approach

History

Establish whether there have been previous attacks, and find out if there are associated features.

Ask about precipitating and relieving factors. Find out sexual and contraceptive habits.

Examination

Examine abdomen and loins for tenderness. Pelvic examination if indicated. Rectal examination in men.

Investigations

Mid-stream urine specimen (MSU) for culture and microscopy (essential in children, adult men and pregnant women).
Intravenous pyelogram (IVP) after treatment in adult men and recurrent infections in women.

Management

Copious fluids by mouth may be the only treatment necessary. Analgesics may be required.

Antibiotics should not be started before obtaining MSU specimen. Initial antibiotics of choice are trimethoprim, co-trimoxazole or nitrofurantoin.

Children and adult males should be referred to a specialist for further investigation. Recurrent 'cystitis' in adult women may require exclusion of precipitating factors and administration of prophylactic antibacterial drugs after intercourse, or at night.

Pain in the Back

Backache is common and disabling. The causes are legion and often unclear and most cases recover spontaneously. Nevertheless, it is a condition of great economic importance to the individual, to industry and to the state.

Common causes

Muscle and ligamentous injury is usually associated with lifting, twisting and sudden movement.
Postural backache due to prolonged standing or sitting in unsuitable positions, common in drivers and typists.

Less common causes

Prolapsed invertebral disc (PID) with low back pain and sciatica.

Bone pain secondary to osteoporosis, malignancy or infection.
Osteoarthritis in the elderly or after trauma.
Chronic depressive illness.
Malingering.

Pitfalls

- In PID, sciatica may occur without lumbago.
- Low back pain occurring for the first time after 50 years of age should be regarded with suspicion.
- Renal lesions or intra-abdominal conditions may produce referred pain in the back.
- Retention of urine in association with PID implies a central prolapse and demands urgent surgical intervention.

Approach

History

Establish the site, mode of onset, severity, radiation and duration of pain. Find out the precipitating and relieving factors and associated symptoms—e.g. urinary, abdominal.

Examination

Watch out for gait, mobility of spine, climbing on couch, and establish if there is local tenderness.
  Examine on straight leg-raising and femoral stretch, and establish tone, power, sensation, reflexes.
  Examine abdomen, general condition and pulse rate (PR) if indicated.

Investigation

Nil in acute cases
If persistent take full blood count (FBC), ESR, biochemical profile (including serum acid phosphatase), serum electrophoresis, urinalysis.
X-ray examination of lumbar spine with or without chest after severe pain has settled (no urgency required).

Management

Insist on strict rest on a firm surface, e.g. bed, floor, and give analgesics and local heat. Possibly give muscle relaxants. Laxatives are often required.

Most 'acute backs' will settle within 3–4 weeks on proper rest. Physiotherapy has a place in the rehabilitation phase of the 'acute back' and in the 'chronic back'. Manipulation may be helpful in the absence of positive neurological signs.

A few patients will require hospital admission for proper rest, epidural injection or surgery.

Subsequent attention to obesity, posture, working and living conditions is important if recurrence is to be avoided.

Pain in the Neck

A 'pain in the neck' is used colloquially to describe someone or something which represents chronic irritation and annoyance.

Common causes

Acute torticollis. Usually occurs in young adults during sleep.
Injury to muscles and ligaments e.g. whiplash in road traffic accident.
Cervical spondylosis.
Osteoarthritis or subluxation of the apophyseal joints in middle-aged and elderly people.

Less common causes

Prolapsed intervertebral disc (usually C6–C7).
Generalised conditions e.g. rheumatoid arthritis, ankylosing spondylitis.
Bone pain which is secondary to Paget's disease, malignancy and infection.

Pitfalls

● Remember to consider the neck as a source of pain presenting in the shoulder and arm.

- Because there is little space in the spinal canal at cervical level minor disc protrusions or tiny osteophytes can impinge on the cord or the vertebral arteries.
- Subluxation of the atlanto-axial joint in rheumatoid arthritis can lead to impingement of the odontoid process onto the cervical cord.

Approach

History

Establish site, mode of onset, severity, radiation and duration of pain. Find out precipitating and relieving factors, and associated symptoms—e.g. sensory, motor, joint pains, vertebrobasilar insufficiency.

Examination

Examine neck, posture, mobility for local tenderness, and examine shoulders and arms. Do neurological and/or general examination if indicated.

Investigation

Nil in acute cases.
If persistent. FBC, ESR, biochemical profile, electrophoresis, urinalysis.
X-ray examination of cervical spine (special views may be required, check with radiologist).

Management

Rest, preferably in a soft collar and give analgesics and local heat. Physiotherapy, manipulation or traction may be helpful if available. Local steroid injections are employed by some doctors. Cervical myelopathy demands urgent referral.

Suspicion of neoplasm, infection, serious trauma or an unsatisfactory response to simple treatment requires referral.

Recurrence is common, especially in mechanical lesions of the lower cervical intervertebral joints. It is worth advising the patient accordingly and keeping a soft collar available.

Vaginal Discharge and Irritation

Vaginal discharge is a common nuisance which causes a great deal of discomfort and anxiety to women in their reproductive years.

Common causes

Excessive physiological secretion during pregnancy, ovulation, pre-menstrually, while on the pill, or caused by 'erosion'.
Monilia with pruritus and soreness, often thick and white discharge.
Trichomonas causing soreness and intertrigo, often frothy and yellowish discharge.
Non-specific vaginitis (NSV) often has unpleasant smell due to *Gardnerella vaginalis*.

Less common causes

Venereal disease. Chlamydia (NSU), gonorrhoea, herpes genitalis.
Malignancy usually with bloodstained discharge.
Opportunist infections such as IUCD, post-partum or post gynaecological surgery, retained tampons or other foreign bodies.
Atrophic vaginitis (oestrogen deficiency) in post-menopausal women.

Pitfalls

- It is very difficult to exclude venereal disease in a woman, especially if it is co-existing with a vaginal infection. If in doubt, refer to a medical genitourinary clinic.

Approach

History

Establish whether there are pruritus, smell, need for protective wear and ask about sexual, contraceptive and menstrual history. Establish whether there is pain or discomfort.

Examination

Abdominal and pelvic examination. Distinguish between vaginitis, cervicitis and vulvitis.

Investigation

Urinalysis for sugar
Take cervical and vaginal swabs in transport medium
Take charcoal swabs from urethra, cervix and rectum if gonorrhoea
is suspected
Take a cervical smear (opportunity for screening).

Management

Give advice about hygiene, avoiding scented soaps, nylon pants,
tights, bath salts, deodorants, etc., and give specific treatment—e.g.
metronidazole for trichomonas, NSV, antifungal agent for monilia;
antibiotics for chlamydia and gonorrhoea; and local oestrogens for
atrophic vaginitis.

Arrange referral for: resistant or recurrent discharge; suspicion of
sexually transmitted disease; and suspicion of malignancy.

Abnormal Vaginal Bleeding

This term covers many conditions, including intermenstrual bleeding, postcoital bleeding, menorrhagia, polymenorrhoea and metropathia haemorrhagica. Some complications of early pregancy are
also included.

Common causes

Contraceptive pill problems especially spotting and breakthrough
bleeding.
Threatened abortion with vaginal bleeding with or without lower
abdominal pain.
Cervical erosion or polyp which is the commonest cause of intermenstrual and postcoital bleeding.
Hormonal imbalance, which may cause anything from amenorrhoea
to metropathia.
Fibroids, often asymptomatic, may cause menorrhagia.

Less common causes

Malignancy of cervix or corpus uteri.
Abnormal pregnancy—ectopic, hydatidiform mole.

71

Endometriosis is often associated with dysmenorrhoea and dyspareunia.

Pitfalls

- It is most important to clarify the position regarding contraception and the possibility of pregnancy.
- It is easy to confuse a carcinoma of the uterus with dysfunc-
tional uterine haemorrhage.
- Do *not* rely on a negative cervical smear if clinically suspicious
of malignancy.

Approach

History

Establish nature, type and pattern of bleeding (menstrual chart may
help), and ask about any associated features such as pain, tiredness,
symptoms of pregnancy. Take sexual and contraceptive history.

Examination

Abdominal and pelvic examination for tenderness, masses, discharge and inspection of cervix.

Investigation

Take a cervical smear.
Take cervical and vaginal swabs if indicated.
Pregnancy test if indicated.
Take haemoglobin estimation.

Management

Reassurance alone may be all that is required, but if not give
specific treatment—e.g. change of contraceptive pill; cyclical hormone therapy; or rest for threatened abortion.
   Arrange referral for: suspected malignancy; endometriosis; large
or symptomatic fibroids; inevitable, incomplete abortion; or ectopic
pregnancy (urgent admission).

Dyspareunia

Dyspareunia may be superficial or deep and due entirely to organic or psychological causes, but commonly both factors will be present.

Common causes

Vulvovaginitis from any cause.
Trauma at first intercourse or postepisiotomy.
Psychosexual problems are often associated with vaginismus.

Less common causes

Pelvic inflammatory disease including cervicitis.
Endometriosis.
Malignancy.

Pitfalls

- Failure to take an adequate history may lead to inappropriate referral and even unnecessary operation.
- It is usually wise to exclude organic causes even if there are obvious psychosexual problems present.

Approach

History

Establish menstrual and obstetric history. Take psychosexual and contraceptive history and find out about associated features.

Examination

During abdominal and pelvic examinations note response to examination and take opportunity to clarify history.

Investigations

Cervical and vaginal swabs should be taken if indicated.
Take a cervical smear (opportunity for screening).

Management

Give advice about nature of problem, and give specific treatment where possible and psychosexual counselling if appropriate.

Arrange referral for pelvic inflammatory disease; endometriosis; and major sexual problems.

Palpitations

Palpitations are distressing and often worrying to patients because in the lay mind they are inevitably associated with heart disease.

Common causes

Paroxysmal supraventricular tachycardia (SVT) which usually occurs in healthy adults.
Anxiety state—fear, hyperventilation.
Ventricular extrasystoles (VE) often described as extra beats or missed beats.

Less common causes

Paroxysmal atrial fibrillation (PAF): patients are usually over 50 years of age.
Thyrotoxicosis must be excluded.
Other cardiac arrythmias that are usually associated with heart disease.

Pitfalls

- It is important to act decisively and reassure the patient confidently if heart disease can be excluded.
- Conversely, it is important not to reassure the patient if the diagnosis is uncertain and further investigation is indicated.
- Atrial fibrillation may be the only evidence of thyrotoxicosis, especially in the elderly.

Approach

History

Establish the nature, duration and regularity of palpitations, and

74

find out the relationship to possible trigger factors—exercise, meals, smoking, alcohol, tea, coffee, anxiety. Also find out about associated features such as dyspnoea, angina, faintness. See if there are features of thyrotoxicosis.

Examination

Check pulse rate and rhythm and blood pressure; ventricular extrasystoles are abolished by exertion, but paroxysmal atrial fibrillation is not.

Check cardiovascular and respiratory system and take thyroid function tests.

Investigation

ECG (during attack if possible).
Take thyroid function tests, if indicated.
Chest x-ray examination.

Management

Give advice about smoking, drinking, tea, coffee, etc. reassure strongly if indicated. Apply vagal stimulation (eyeball pressure or carotid massage) for SVT.

Give β-blockers for SVT, thyrotoxicosis and give specific treatment for cardiac failure, ischaemic heart disease and valvular heart disease.

Arrange referral for elucidation of arrhythmia, specific anti-arrhythmic medication, and cardioversion.

Hyperventilation

This is a common reaction to pain or anxiety, but occasionally is a pointer to serious underlying disease.

Common causes

Anxiety.
Response to pain, which may cause paraesthesiae and tetany.

75

Less common causes

Respiratory disease such as emphysema, pneumonia, asthma.
Diabetic keto-acidosis.
Aspirin overdose.

Pitfalls

● Failure to consider underlying disease if hyperventilation persists.

Approach

History

Establish facts about onset, precipitating factors and associated features.

Examination

This should be general (for reassurance).

Investigation

Not usually required.

Management

A calm, relaxed manner will reassure the patient. Suggest rebreathing from paper or plastic bag, and manage as appropriate for any underlying condition.

Insomnia

The amount of sleep which people require varies enormously from person to person. If they feel well and function normally then the duration and quality of sleep is adequate for that person.

Common causes

Shiftwork
External factors such as noise, snoring partner, uncomfortable bed.

Anxiety/tension often with a long history of difficulty in falling asleep.
Hypnotic dependence developing tolerance to sedatives.
Ageing. Sleep patterns change in the elderly.
Pain and discomfort.

Less common causes

Depression is classically associated with early waking.

Pitfalls

- Do not prescribe hypnotics before exploring underlying causes.
- Beware of attempted suicide by using an overdose of hypnotics.
- There is a danger of missing a depressive illness with serious results.

Approach

History

Ask about the pattern of sleep disturbance and previous sleep problems. Establish past psychiatric history, and find out if there are any social and emotional problems. Also find out about physical problems.

Examination

Examine if necessary to exclude physical disease.

Investigation

Usually unnecessary.

Management

Explain and reassure, and, give counselling if appropriate. Also, give advice about relaxation and promotion of natural sleep—e.g. hot bath, hot drink, reading.

Suggest altering environment where possible, and give specific treatment for pain with analgesics; depression with antidepressants.

Hypnotics should be prescribed in small quantities for short periods only and barbiturates avoided.

13. PROFESSIONAL SERVICES

As the doctor of first contact, the GP sees a number of patients who are not ill but who have consulted either for planned or preventive care—e.g. family planning, antenatal care, immunisations or for certificates of one sort or another which only a doctor can provide.

Obviously if the practice provides a high-quality service in health education and preventive medicine it is of great benefit to both patients and doctors. Less obviously of benefit to the doctor is the provision of administrative services to his or her patients, but a helpful and considerate attitude by the doctor can strengthen his relationship with the patient thus helping it to withstand future strains more easily.

In this chapter we try to cover the main areas where patients consult not for illness *per se*, but for advice or for preventive or administrative action.

Abortion Counselling

The large majority of patients who consult have already made up their minds and do not want counselling but referral to an appropriate agency.

When others seem to be speaking for the patient she should be interviewed by herself to find out her real views.

The doctor should gather all the relevant facts before deciding what course to take.

(1) Refer for NHS abortion

  ● the views of the consultant the patient sees will determine whether abortion is carried out or not
  ● if carried out it is free
  ● best done before 12–13 weeks' gestation but can be done up to 20 weeks or more with prostaglandins.

78

(2) Refer for private abortion

- abortion will almost certainly be carried out
- costs £100 or so
- in most areas it is likely to be safer, both in terms of mortality and morbidity, than an NHS abortion.

(3) Advise the patient to seek a second opinion from another doctor

- the doctor is supposed to do this if he or she has an ethical objection to referring patients for abortion.

(4) Advise the patient to consider proceeding with the pregnancy and keeping the baby or having it adopted.

- this advice is most unlikely to be heeded unless the patient is already working towards this decision herself.

The doctor's personal beliefs concerning abortion will determine the outcome of the consultation rather than any considered interpretation of the Abortion Act.

Modern abortion techniques, carried out before 12–13 weeks' gestation, do not appreciably impair future fertility. Patients who are refused abortion and go to term are more likely to suffer severe psychological disturbance than those who have abortions.

Antenatal Care

In 80% of cases, care is shared by GP and specialist obstetrician. Unless there are problems the bulk of the antenatal care is carried out by the GP with the hospital seeing the patient for booking, at 32 and/or 36 weeks and at term.

In 20% of cases care is provided solely by the GP, who also accepts the responsibility for backing up the midwife who supervises the delivery. Normally only those patients who, as far as one can predict, are going to have problem-free pregnancies and confinements are considered suitable for this type of care.

Objectives

(1) To prepare, educate, inform and help the expectant mother

to achieve an enjoyable pregnancy, a safe delivery and a normal baby.

(2) To create and maintain good relations between the mother and the practice team (receptionist, health visitor, midwife and GP).

(3) To collaborate closely with local specialist obstetric and paediatric units.

Practice organisation

This should ensure that:

(1) Antenatal care routines are clearly understood by patient and practice team.

(2) There are good shared records.

(3) There are speedy lines of communication with specialist services when difficulties arise.

(4) There are systems to keep late bookings to a minimum and to follow up defaulters and irregular attenders.

(5) There are clearly defined obstetric, medical and social risk factors which will lead to referral to specialist units.

An overall plan

Regular attendance is easier for patient and practice to follow, but flexibility may be necessary in individual cases. Present antenatal routines are outline in Table 13.1.

Problems within this plan that should be considered include the following:

- Do all patients need iron and/or folic acid supplements and, if not, who does?
- What is the value of routinely listening to fetal hearts?
- Can antenatal care be humanised so that patients get time to talk about their worries rather than get processed mechanically?
- Why should patients be seen so often when likely pick-up rates for abnormalities, especially in the first 30 weeks, are so low? Would being seen at 8–12, 20, 26, 30, 34, 36 weeks and then weekly to term be as good?

Table 13.1 *Present antenatal routines for patient and practice*

Consultation	Practice staff or doctor	Doctor

Booking (8–12 weeks)	Fill in form FP24 or 24A
	Fill in personal details on cooperation card
	Weight
	Urinalysis (albumin/glucose)
	Blood pressure
	Fill in forms for:
	  – Hb
	  – ABO and Rhesus
	  – Rubella antibodies
	  – VDRL
	  – MSU
	  – Electrophoresis for abnormal Hb in women of African, Indian or Mediterranean extraction
	Take blood specimens
		Full medical history
		Menstrual history
		Calculate expected date of delivery
		Past gynaecological history
		Past obstetric history
		Physical examination, including breasts, CVS, abdomen
		Anti-smoking propaganda
		Pro-breastfeeding propaganda
		Decide form and place of antenatal care and delivery
		Discuss patient worries/fears
		Fill in cooperation card

4-weekly (until 28 weeks)	Weight Blood pressure Urinalysis (albumin/glucose) Start routine iron/folic acid	Note when fetal movements felt Check fundus Discuss patient worries/fears
2-weekly (28–36 weeks) then weekly to term	Weight Blood pressure Urinalysis (albumin/glucose) Encourage care of breasts Arrange for parentcraft, relaxation classes, etc	Check fundus/fetal heart Confirm fetal position Check expected date of delivery Discuss patient worries/fears At 30 and 36 weeks check Hb, Rhesus antibodies if appropriate At 36 weeks check head engaged
Postnatal (6–8 weeks after delivery)	Weight Blood pressure Urinalysis (albumin/glucose) Send off completed form FP24 or 24A	Examine breasts and pelvis Cervical smear if indicated Discuss contraception Follow-up any antenatal or labour problems Complete form FP24 or 24A Complete form FP1001 or 1002 Inquire about baby's progress

Alphafetoprotein screening is now being carried out in many areas:

- Blood is best taken at 16–18 weeks (not before 16).
- Screening picks up 80–90% of fetuses with open spina bifida and anencephalus.
- Couples must understand that a normal result does not guarantee a normal fetus.
- Only worth doing in patients who would consider termination should the result prove to be positive.

Amniocentesis should be offered to all pregnant women over the age of 36. It can pick up chromosomal abnormalities, e.g. Down's syndrome, open neural tube defects (fluid alphafetoprotein levels measured), and male fetuses at risk of a sex-linked disorder—i.e. if risk of haemophilia it could show that the fetus was male but not whether that male would actually get haemophilia or not. There is the risk of spontaneous abortion in 1% of cases, and it does not guarantee a normal fetus and should not be carried out unless termination would be considered should an abnormality be discovered.

Cervical Cytology

Smears detect dysplastic changes at the cervical squamocolumnar junction so allowing early treatment to prevent the development of invasive carcinoma.

In about 30% of cases dysplasia, after an interval of 8–10 years, will progress to invasive carcinoma. Routine 5-yearly smears will therefore pick up the large majority of cases in time for effective treatment.

The first smear should be taken about age 20–25, usually after sexual activity has begun. Under certain circumstances a fee is claimable (see the Red Book).

To take a smear:

- using a speculum, lubricated only with water, completely expose the cervix;
- with wooden spatula take a firm scrape of the squamo columnar junction through a full 360°;
- spread the material obtained thinly, to form a monocellular layer, on a glass slide; and
- fix the slide material with a solution of 95% alcohol.

A practice screening policy (on whom, when, how often, by whom?) helps all partners and staff to give consistent advice. If a patient requests smears more often than seems appropriate then her reasons should be explored and advice given.

A well-trained practice nurse can run an intrapractice smear clinic with cases either self-referred, referred by the doctors or selected from the age–sex register.

If a smear is abnormal then the report will usually contain suggestions for appropriate action:

- mild cases (grade III) require repeat smears in 6–12 months;
- severer cases or persistent mild cases require gynaecological referral for colposcopy; and
- trichomonas or thrush infection noted on a smear probably does not require treatment unless the patient has symptoms.

Contraception

Most patients who come for contraceptive advice are either well established on a method or have clear ideas about which method they want to use.

If general advice is wanted or if the doctor does not think the method they are using or wish to use is likely to be safest or most reliable for them then remember the following:

(1) Discuss the advantages and disadvantages of all the feasible methods.

(2) The acceptability of the method to the couple may be as important as any medical consideration.

(3) Method safety studies show that:

- vasectomy is the safest and most effective method of contraception at any age;
- female sterilisation is better than any reversible method used for the same number of years;
- a barrier method combined with early abortion if unplanned pregnancy occurs is safe and effective;
- deaths from the pill increase greatly after the age of 35; and
- any method is safer than none.

Effective long-term use depends to a large degree on patient confidence and satisfaction with the standard of care they are receiving. Good care includes the following.

(1) An up-to-date well-informed doctor who can fit both diaphragms and coils.

(2) An integrated screening programme so that rubella status is checked in nullips; 5-yearly smears are performed on all patients; and all patients are offered a leaflet or advice on self-examination of the breasts.

(3) A special contraceptive record card is kept in the notes.

(4) An intrapractice family planning clinic either run by the doctor or a family planning-trained practice nurse who can carry out pill, coil and diaphragm checks as well as fitting diaphragms and taking smears.

Fees may be claimed annually on forms FP 1001 or FP 1002 (see the Red Book).

The combined pill

The combined pill is virtually 100% effective and best used (1) below the age of 35, (2) when couple wish to be certain no pregnancy will occur, and (3) if woman suffers from any condition which the pill will benefit or relieve.

All varieties have 50 μg of oestrogen or less and for practical purposes the choice of oestrogen or progestogen in the pill is unimportant.

Up to 3 days after unprotected intercourse two Ovran or Eugynon 50 tablets taken stat and again in 12 hours may provide postcoital contraception.

Absolute contraindictions

The combined pill should not be used when any of the following conditions are present:

(1) Over 35-year-old women who smoke.

(2) Intravascular thrombosis including any condition predisposing to thromboembolism.

(3) Heart diseases including septal defects, mitral stenosis.

(4) Impaired liver function/porphyria/gallstones.

(5) Possible sex hormone-dependent tumours.

(6) Undiagnosed abnormal vaginal bleeding.

(7) Pregnancy.
(8) Pre-existing neuro-ophthalmic disorders.
(9) Pituitary dysfunction.
(10) Any condition that deteriorated appreciably in pregnancy.
(11) Recent hydatidiform mole.

Relative contraindictions

Over-35 or over-30 if woman is smoker or has any other risk factor, e.g.:
Moderate hypertension.
Obesity.
Diabetes.
Migraine.
Lactation.
Depressive states.
Epilepsy.
Oligomenorrhoea.
Otosclerosis.
Liver disorder.
Renal disease.

NB In these cases the combined pill represents a lesser risk than pregnancy, should no other method be acceptable or sufficiently effective, though special supervision is required.

Possible adverse effects

Minor side effects (nausea, irritability, breast tenderness, etc) are common and usually disappear within a few cycles. As with loss of libido and depression, headaches including migraine are as likely to be improved as worsened by the pill though if headaches are precipitated by the pill or migraine worsened then the pill should be stopped.

Rarer more serious risks to health include thromboembolism, circulatory diseases, hypertension and gallstones—their incidence can be decreased by preprescription screening of users and careful follow-up monitoring.

Adverse effects do not include the development of diabetes, neoplasms or infertility.

Incidence reduction

Reduction of incidence of menorrhagia, dysmenorrhoea, premenstrual tension, mid-cycle pain, endometriosis, iron deficiency anaemia, benign breast disease, carcinoma ovary, acne (in most patients).

Starting the pill

(1) Before prescribing the pill assess risk factors and exclude contraindications from the history.
(2) Check blood pressure, note weight, institute screening programme, consider performing vaginal examination (do not insist if patient appears at all reluctant).
(3) Explain how the pill works and how to take it (a leaflet may be helpful).
(4) Prescribe a low dose pill, e.g. Ovranette, Microgynon, and ask patient to return in three months.

Follow-up

(1) After initial 3 months patient should be seen 6 monthly with blood pressure checked at every visit.
(2) Review any problems or worries about pill use.
(3) If breakthrough bleeding is occurring the most likely remedy in the first instance is to increase the progestogen (to Ovran 30 or Eugynon 30).
(4) If pill not suiting the woman change from one preparation to another; this does not appear to lead to any loss of protection.
(5) If patient wishes to delay a period then she should take packets without a break.

The progestogen only pill (mini-pill)

The mini-pill is effective and best used in over-35s who do not wish sterilisation and while breast feeding.

Absolute contraindications

A recent hydatidiform mole and a history of ectopic pregnancy.

Relative contraindications

Hypertension, history of thromboembolism and risk factors for ectopic pregnancy.

Side effects

Bleeding abnormalities and breast soreness, but serious adverse effects are rare. If pregnancy occurs while on this pill then it may be ectopic.

Starting and follow-up

As for the combined pill.

The intrauterine contraceptive device (IUCD) or coil

The IUCD is effective and best used as an alternative to the pill for those women who have at least one child; as an alternative to sterilisation for women coming off the pill; and for the forgetful.

Absolute contraindications

Pregnancy, history of ectopic pregnancy, active pelvic inflammation, undiagnosed irregular genital tract bleeding.

Relative contraindications

History of pelvic infection, nulliparity, menorrhagia/anaemia, previous caesarean section, bleeding tendency/anticoagulation, abnormalities of the uterine cavity.

Adverse effects
- If there is pregnancy it may be ectopic.
- Pelvic inflammation.
- Uterine bleeding and pain.
- Expulsion of the device.
- Perforation of the uterus.

Insertion techniques should be learned from training at a recognised centre. A GP who advises a patient to have a coil fitted, but does not fit coils, may refer the patient to a family planning clinic or hospital and claim the FP 1001 fee rather than the FP 1002. If pregancy occurs with a coil *in situ* the patient should be referred to an obstetrician for removal of the coil.

Remove the coil by pulling threads with sponge forceps, downwards in direction of the long axis of the cervix. Best removed just after a period.

A coil inserted up to 7 days after unprotected intercourse will provide effective postcoital contraception because it interferes with implantation of the blastocyst.

Diaphragm and chemicals

The diaphragm is effective if used properly by a well-motivated woman. May be used in any age group by women who cannot or do not wish to take the pill.

There are no adverse effects and it may give protection against cervical cancer.

Spermicide must always be used and although the diaphragm may be fitted at any time before intercourse (extra spermicide if more than 6 hours before) it should not be removed until 6 hours after.

Training in fitting should be given by the practice family planning nurse or doctor.

The sheath

The sheath is much under-rated, being potentially an effective, cheap and easy to use method.

Primary reasons for failure include the following.

(1) When it is not used on every conceivable occasion.
(2) When there is penetration before the sheath is put on.
(3) Failure to unroll the sheath to entire length or to leave sufficient space at the tip to act as ejaculate reservoir.
(4) Failure to withdraw while penis is still erect.

Sterilisation

In either partner sterilisation is safer and more effective than using any reversible method for the same number of years, but it should not be entered into lightly. It must be emphasised to the couple that for all practical purposes the procedures are irreversible.

There must be a full measure of counselling about medical and social factors and their implications for the future.

If all else is equal vasectomy is prefereable to female sterilisation because it is easier to perform and safer.

Prenatal and Genetic Counselling

Advice may be sought before starting a family, either because of the possible risks that familial disease might pose to the baby or because of worries about pregnancy itself

Specialist guidance may be sought on the risk of a disease or disability affecting the baby. The consultation may also be used to discuss basic arrangements for pregnancy care; good health rules for the mother-to-be; any fears or worries that may exist. If not known, rubella status should be ascertained.

Any patient who has an abnormal baby should be offered the opportunity of taking specialist genetic advice on the likely risk of recurrence in any other pregnancies.

Assessment of a Child's Development

Intensive developmental screening is of unproved value. Doctors who hold regular intrapractice developmental clinics argue that giving support and advice to parents is as important as the detection of abnormalities.

Whether a formal practice screening policy exists or not every GP should, at any consultation concerning a child, be looking for and recognising defects outside the range of normal. A GP should also be able to make a reliable appraisal of a child's development and give sound guidance in answer to parents' questions.

Development

A child's development is of increasing complexity while growth is increasing. It takes place in various different ways (locomotion, manipulation, use of eyes and ears, speech, etc) and though all babies follow the same sequence of development the rate varies from child to child. Even the same child does not develop at a constant rate but in lulls and spurts.

Uniformly retarded development implies mental retardation or severe emotional deprivation. Slowness in one particular field is not a sign of retardation but may be due to a family trait; lack of stimulation; or physical disease.

Progress depends on the maturing of the central nervous system and so cannot be accelerated by outside stimulation. On the other hand, illness and environmental factors may retard it.

Assessment

This requires answers to the following questions:

(1) Is this child developing normally?
(2) Is the child's behaviour appropriate for its age?
(3) Does the child still exhibit signs of earlier behaviour which by now should have gone?
(4) Are there any abnormal signs?

Infants with major abnormalities or abnormalities which might have important consequences should be referred to a (developmental) paediatrician. So should any infant which has not reached an important milestone at the age when most infants would have been

Table 13.2 *Developmental delay at various age limits*

Referral age	Behaviour
6 months	Head still wobbly Fists clenched Not reaching with hands
12 months	Not able to sit without support Not able to take weight on legs Not transferring between hands Not looking Not listening
18 months	Not walking alone Not vocalising Still casting objects Still mouthing
24 months	Not saying a single word Not showing any imagination or imitation in play Lack of interest

90

expected to. The age when most infants should possess an ability is known as the limit age. Some important limit ages are shown in Table 13.2.

Discussion of Whooping Cough Vaccination

Since concern over the safety of pertussis vaccination was first voiced in 1974 the percentage of children under 2 who are vaccinated has dropped from 78% to 38% and there has been a major rise in the incidence of whooping cough (102 000 cases notified in the 1977–79 epidemic).

Parents may seek advice before having their baby vaccinated. Some points are worth making:

(1) Whooping cough is a serious disease causing death (28 in 1977–79) as well as an unknown number of cases of brain and lung damage.

(2) Of children below the age of 2 with whooping cough, 10% have to be admitted to hospital.

(3) Medical treatment is unsatisfactory.

(4) Vaccination is over 90% effective.

(5) Minor reactions to vaccination (irritability, pyrexia, sore arm, vomiting) occur in up to 10% of cases and resolve within 24–48 hours.

(6) In children who are potential febrile-fitters a vaccine-induced fever may provoke a fit but fits are common at this age anyway and there is no evidence that the vaccine causes fits directly.

(7) The vaccine does cause some cases of serious brain damage. If all 600 000 children born in Britain each year undergo a full course of pertussis vaccination then six will have a severe reaction and be left with a permanent disability (75% of the children developing serious reactions will do so within 24 hours of vaccination).

Contraindications to vaccination

● Where there is a history of fits in the child or close family history of fits (parents, sibs, grandparents).

● Where there is any abnormality of the central nervous system.

- Where there has been a severe reaction to a previous dose of triple vaccine (no more pertussis, but continue with the others).
- When the child has an acute illness with a fever (wait until better and then vaccinate).

For normal children, without contraindications, the benefits of vaccination outweigh the risks, though only the parents can decide what is best for their child. If the doctor's own children have been vaccinated, telling the parents so will be more useful than making any number of medical points.

It is vital that the entire practice (partners, health visitors, nurses) follow the same guidelines for advising parents. Team members may well benefit from intrapractice teaching or discussion on this topic.

Immunisation for a Child

In many practices routine immunisation are carried out by the practice nurse and not the doctor. The doctor remains responsible for the nurse's actions and must ensure that she is fully trained and competent. Regular teaching sessions are necessary.

Schedule

- Diphtheria/tetanus/pertussis (triple) and polio immunisation at 3, $4\frac{1}{2}$, $8\frac{1}{2}$–11 months.
- Measles immunisation at 15 months
- Diphtheria/tetanus and polio immunisation at $4\frac{1}{2}$ years.
- If pertussis is not wanted or is contraindicated then give diphtheria/tetanus immunisation.
- In the event of a whooping cough outbreak a crash regimen of three doses of triple at monthly intervals from the age of 3 months may be given. A diphtheria/tetanus booster then has to be given at 12–18 months.

Contraindications

Diphtheria. No contraindications but should not be given to people over the age of 10 years unless they are Schick-positive.
Tetanus. None, but once the basic course is complete there should be at least one year between boosters.

Pertussis. See p. 91. Additionally should not be given to any child over the age of 3 years.

Polio. Immunological dysfunction; malignant disease; steroid therapy; immunosuppressant therapy; radiotherapy; past history of adverse reaction to penicillin; within 3 weeks of another live vaccine; pregnancy (in adults). If diarrhoea and vomiting or an acute febrile illness are present vaccination should be postponed.

Measles. As for polio but also including active tuberculosis; allergy to egg; history or family history of convulsions.

Administration

See Table 13.3.

Waiting for babies to be brought for immunisations is not enough. Use of the age–sex register, or a card index system, allows a record to be kept of each baby vaccinated—those who are shown to have missed vaccinations can then be actively followed up by the health visitor.

Table 13.3   *Administration of vaccine for immunisation of child*

Vaccine	Dose	Adverse effects	Notes
Triple	0.5 ml × 3 i.m. or deep s.c.	Transient local erythema and tenderness Restlessness and irritability in 24 hours after vaccination Occasional screaming fits Rarely encephalopathy	If only first dose given then two doses at about six months' interval needed If only first two doses given then third will probably be effective up to 12 months after the second
Polio (Sabin)	3 drops × 3 oral	Rarely vaccine related paralysis in recipients or contacts	Unvaccinated parents of a child being immunised should also be offered immunisation
Measles	0.5 ml i.m. or s.c.	Usually about 8th day with mild cough, cold, rash, pyrexia Rarely high pyrexia and febrile fit Encephalitis in 1 in 1 m cases	Vaccine is quickly killed by ether, alcohol or detergents so wash skin with water only If chronic heart or lung disease give concomitant injection of gammaglobulin into the muscle of the opposite limb

A Letter or Certificate for a Third Party

GPs have access to considerable amounts of information about their patients. They are also considered to be unbiased and truthful in a way that individual patients are not.

A great variety of bodies (employers, Department of Health and Social Security, councils, social services, lawyers and insurance companies) will approach GPs for verification of information that a patient has already given them or for a medical opinion to help them assess a patient's capabilities or needs.

If the approach comes through the patient the following should be remembered.

(1) Implied consent is given for the release of confidential information.

(2) In many cases a fee may be asked for but, depending on individual circumstances, this is often waived.

(3) If a fee is payable by the official body, provided that they have approached the doctor directly, the patient should be advised to ask them to write.

(4) Even when a request seems frivolous or vexatious, before refusing out of hand remember that the patient may be trapped between two powerful bodies, *viz* the GP and the third party, and the GP is likely to be the more sympathetic. Giving the patients what they need and then writing strong letters to the bodies concerned may be the best line of action.

If the approach comes directly from a third party the following applies.

(1) The patient's explicit written authority for the release of confidential information is necessary.

(2) Even if there is written authority, should it seem possible that the patient does not appreciate the implications of what is going to be disclosed he or she should be interviewed first.

(3) Keep a record of the fee owed so that a payment reminder may be sent if the bill is not met in good time.

A Medical Check-Up

It is transparently obvious to the laymen that a check-up is a good thing to have and so check-ups are gaining in popularity. Problems posed in practice are as follows:

- Check-ups are time-consuming procedures.
- There is no objective evidence that they are of any real benefit.
- There is no extra fee for service under the NHS, and no private fee is allowable.
- There is no agreed standard programme.
- There are no special NHS records for the exercise.

A request for a check-up may be a cry for much more than a physical examination and personal and family psychosocial matters should be explored.

While the GP would be within his rights to refuse to perform a check-up perhaps the opportunity could at least be used to discuss personal health risk habits and to check the blood pressure.

Overseas Travel Advice

Prospective travellers will consult primarily for vaccinations, but some may come to ask for prescriptions for travel sickness pills, antidiarrhoeal mixtures or even calamine lotion. Do not prescribe, but advise that such medicines may be bought from the chemist.

The DHSS booklet '*Notice to Travellers—Health Protection*' may be obtained free from the DHSS and given to each overseas traveller.

General advice

(1) Never trust the cleanliness of drinking water unless sure it has been boiled and never drink milk that has not been pasteurised or boiled.

(2) Bottled or aerated waters are safe to drink.

(3) Do not eat unwashed vegetables or fruit unless they have an intact detachable cover—e.g. oranges.

(4) Check safety of all swimming areas before bathing.

(5) Take out adequate medical insurance cover.

(6) If ill for any length of time seek reliable medical advice (bank, embassy, airline will give you a safe contact).

(7) Take a small medical kit containing paracetamol, Codis (for diarrhoea), antifungal powder, antiseptic cream, band-aid plasters, antimalarials.

Table 13.4 *Vaccinations needed in various parts of the world (view with Table 13.5)*

Area	Vaccinations (* mandatory)
South Europe	Polio
Central and South America	Yellow fever*, typhoid, polio
Middle East	Typhoid, cholera, polio
North Africa	Typhoid, cholera, polio
Central, East and West Africa	Yellow fever*, typhoid, polio
South Africa	Typhoid, polio
Indian subcontinent	Typhoid, polio
South-East Asia and China	Typhoid, polio

Immunisation

Many travellers do not consult early enough to allow for optimal spacing of vaccinations—a rapid scheme may be used though less effective immunity is gained.

Travellers to northern Europe, North America, Japan, Australia and New Zealand require no particular immunisation though

Table 13.5 *Vaccine programme*

Yellow fever (live)	Given at special centres One injection gives immunity for 10 years Not within two weeks of polio or gammaglobulin
Typhoid (killed)	Two doses at 4–6 week interval Three-yearly boosters if still exposed to risk
Cholera (killed)	Two doses at 1–4 weeks' interval Six-monthly booster if still exposed to risk International certificate of vaccination required for entry into some countries
Polio (live)	Three doses at six weeks then six-month intervals Five-yearly booster Not within two weeks of yellow fever or gammaglobulin
Tetanus (toxoid)	Three doses at four weeks then six-month intervals 10 yearly booster
Gammaglobulin	Protects against hepatitis A for up to six months Give four days or so before travel

NB For all vaccinations look up dosage, route of administration, contraindications and side effects, on the label or notes accompanying the vaccine.

96

tetanus booster may be indicated, especially for campers. For other areas of the world check Table 13.4 then Table 13.5 to plan individual programme.

See the Red Book for fees that are claimable from NHS for overseas vaccination. If no fee is claimable or if international certificate required you may charge a private fee (see BMA booklet; establish practice policy).

- For all countries check if tetanus toxoid needed, especially by campers or overland travellers.
- For overland travellers and those going to primitive regions use human normal immunoglobulin (HNIG) for prophylaxis against hepatitis A.
- For travellers (not holidaymakers) to primitive regions give rabies vaccine.
- Smallpox vaccination should not be required by any traveller.

Malaria prophylaxis

Protection is necessary for even a one-day stay in a malaria area. Tablets to be taken one week before travel and continued until 6 weeks after return to UK.

For Africa, Arab states, Pakistan, India (except Eastern India), Pacific islands give Paludrine 200 mg daily or chloroquine 300 mg weekly.

Eastern India, Bangladesh, South East Asia, Central and South America, Papua New Guinea give Maloprim one tablet weekly or Fansidar one tablet weekly (not for pregnant women or those sensitive to sulfas).

Children for doses for each age, see Data Sheet Compendium.

NB Tablets cannot be given on NHS prescription but may be a private prescription or bought, without prescription, at chemist.

Referral for a Second Opinion

In any year up to 20% of persons in Britain are referred by GPs to consultants for their specialist opinion and technical expertise. On average, a GP will write eight referral letters a week and the best ones will be brief and to the point explaining what the problem is, what investigations or treatment has been carried out, why referral is taking place and what is expected from the consultant.

A cardinal ethical rule is that no consultant should see a patient without a GP's referral letter. This still holds true for NHS patients, though many consultants are happy to give their opinion to unreferred patients prepared to pay for the privilege.

In many cases where the GP has not thought of getting a second opinion a patient's request for referral may come as quite a surprise. The doctor may feel upset, hurt, bewildered, rejected or even angry.

The doctor's feelings notwithstanding, the patient's wishes should be calmly explored.

(1) Is the patient unhappy with the doctor's care? If so, in what way?

(2) Does the patient not believe or not accept the diagnosis (or lack of it)?

(3) Are the implications of the diagnosis such that a different opinion is desired?

(4) Does the patient, or relatives, feel that alternative or better treatment is available elsewhere?

Discussion may result in the following.

● The patient's fears or worries being allayed so that the relationship with the doctor is strengthened.

● An improvement in the standard of care or, at the least, the patient's perception of it.

● A reasonable referral instituted, without acrimony, either through the NHS or privately.

● A totally unreasonable request turned down after obviously careful consideration and explanation.

● A recognition that the doctor/patient relationship has totally broken down and that it would be best for the patient to see a different doctor.

For patients who have a habit of constantly seeking second opinions, without paying much attention to the first, the GP must decide whether he can live with this behaviour or whether the patient should be asked to leave his list.

14. EMERGENCIES

Responsibilities

The GP is obliged by the terms of service to provide 24 hour medical care for patients. He or she must also respond to emergency calls for any patients in a practice area if the patient's own doctor is not available.

The GP is *not* obliged to visit on request—only as the occasion demands. Responsibility for the decision is the doctor's.

If the duty is delegated to a doctor who is *not* on the FPC list, the delegating doctor retains responsibility for actions.

Preparation and equipment

The visiting bag

The contents are an individual matter.

Equipment in the car

- Brook airway.
- Spare syringes, path. bottles.
- Oxygen giving set.
- Saline drip set.
- Torch and map of the area.
- List of telephone numbers—hospitals, ambulance, etc.
- Supply of forms, letter paper, etc., in car or bag.

NB Make sure that the car is reliable.

The house

Have a telephone extension in bedroom. Get your line listed as an emergency number. This gives you priority for repairs.

Ideally you need someone in the house to answer the telephone when you are out on a call. If you live alone you will need an answering machine.

Familiarise yourself with telephone procedures.

Telephone answering

Virtually all emergency calls are made by telephone. A kind considerate manner will enable you to get information while keeping the caller happy.

You are not obliged to visit, but if the caller is in a panic, or aggressive, *visit first*. Explain and educate later. If you are going to visit say so early on because this allays anxiety. Advice should be clear and simple.

Encourage the caller to ring back if the situation changes or if worried.

The most important item of information is the patient's *name and address*.

The nature of emergency calls

Several surveys show that most calls are not frivolous.

Young parents who have little knowledge of illness become acutely anxious about symptoms that appear trivial to the doctor. The call may reflect the fact that the family is under stress, or that the extra anxiety cannot be tolerated. It may be used as a weapon. Relatives who do not want to become involved in caring will often pass on responsibility by calling the doctor.

Anxiety in the caller may cause an aggressive manner. Previous contact with unwilling doctors may also cause aggression in an effort to ensure a visit.

Appropriate action

Direct patient to hospital if major trauma, burns or poisoning, call ambulance. Only go yourself if you can do something useful.
Visit if medically indicated or if caller's anxieties and expectations are such that advice will not be tolerated when the problem is discussed on the telephone.
Give advice for simple illnesses where caller is satisfied and intelligent enough to understand instructions.

Principles of management in the home

● A calm methodical approach is vital even if you are cross or worried.

100

- A careful history and examination gets you the information you need as well as having a calming effect on the patient.
- Deciding on correct disposal is more important than making an accurate diagnosis.
- Give clear and simple instructions—written if necessary.
- Educate at every opportunity, but only after you have examined and made your decisions.
- Make careful notes.
- Arrange for any necessary follow-up.

Admissions

Reasons for admission

Where there is a medical necessity and/or social conditions make home care difficult.

When there is abuse of children or elderly, and when admission is demanded by patient or relative (rare).

Responsibility

Having made the decision that an admission is necessary, it is the GP's duty to implement this.

(1) Contact local hospitals: if there is no bed contact consultant. If no help there, contact medical referee of Hospital Bed Bureau (you can get the telephone number from the hospital or district health authority).

(2) Arrange ambulance giving degree of urgency.

(3) Send letter with full information including details of allergies and drug treatment. Be honest about reasons for admission.

Clinical Management

In this book it is not possible to give a complete guide to the management of all emergencies, but some problems which are either unique to general practice, or which present particular problems for the trainee, are as follows.

Paediatric Emergencies

Special problems

- A great many out-of-hours calls are for acute illnesses in children.
- Parents, especially the young and isolated, are very anxious.
- Listen carefully to parents—they are often right about their child, even when you cannot find anything wrong.
- Repeated or unnecessary calls may be due to: excessive anxiety, family stress, child abuse, or low intelligence.
- The clinical condition of children changes rapidly, so always be willing to see the patient again to reassess.

The examination

- Patience and tolerance are needed.
- Small children are calmer if examined on mother's lap.
- All systems must be examined every time. The symptoms of small children are not well localised, e.g. otitis media may be the cause of vomiting.
- Undress the child (take nappy off).

Child abuse

Always be on the lookout for evidence of mental or physical abuse. Abuse is often associated with:

(1) Low birth weight babies.
(2) Babies who have been separated from mother soon after birth.
(3) Young parents.
(4) Social or emotional difficulties.
(5) Frequent attendances at surgery or casualty.
(6) Children with feeding problems, crying and vomiting.

Parents at the end of their tether may be anxious or aggressive.

Potential abuse

If you detect excessive tension ask the parents in a kind and sympathetic way if they sometimes feel violent. Offer maximum support from yourself, the health visitor, or from social services.

If the situation is tense then admit the child to hospital to allow the crisis to cool off.

Established abuse

Admit immediately to hospital, if abuse is established, and inform social services.

The crying child

A crying child is a frequent reason for an emergency call and generates much anxiety in parents and doctor.

Crying of acute onset

Severe crying or screaming in a normally happy child is significant.

Assessment

Find out if crying is associated with being touched or moved, or with defecation or micturation. Does the child draw up legs? Is it episodic? Any recent trauma or illness? Examine carefully—particularly ears, abdomen, genitalia and bones, and test for meningism.

Common causes are:

- Otitis media.
- Abdominal pain—often colic (remember intussusception).
- Osteomyelitis.
- Fracture (remember abuse).
- Strangulated hernia.
- Torsion of testicle.
- Inflamed foreskin—pain on micturition.
- Inflamed perianal area due to diarrhoea.

Management

Treatment of the underlying condition. If no cause is found, child may need admission for observation.

The always crying child

The emergency call is usually because parents have reached the end of their tether. They may be aggressive—'There must be something wrong with him.'

Watch out for potential baby battering.

Assessment

Carefully examine child to reassure parents. Typically the baby is well and gaining weight.

Management

Reassurance and support from you or health visitor. If baby is at risk *admit*.

The feverish child

Other symptoms often indicate the cause of the fever but it is the fever itself that usually worries the parents.

Indications for a visit

(1) If the children are young—especially below 2 years-of-age.
(2) Where there is a very high temperature or history of febrile convulsions.
(3) When the child is excessively drowsy or irritable.
(4) When parents are very anxious.
(5) Where there is no obvious cause or possible serious cause for fever.

Telephone advice

- Reassure—fever is not in itself dangerous.
- Keep the child cool and give plenty of fluids.
- Use aspirin or paracetamol only if the child is irritable.
- Call again if fever persists or is child gets worse.

Assessment and management

Do careful examination of child to find cause and treat accordingly.

If there is a clear risk of a febrile fit, give 0.25 mg/kg rectal, diazepam (Valium).

Do not use antibiotics unless there is a clear indication.

The child with croup

Croup is the symptom complex of an explosive cough, a hoarse voice and stridor. It is caused by acute laryngotracheobronchitis, acute epiglottitis or a foreign body.

Acute largyngotracheobronchitis

It may precede a cold, it is mildly febrile and not very toxic, and there is a pronounced cough with high-pitched stridor.

Acute epiglottitis

Onset is sudden and may be preceded by a sore throat. The child, is very toxic, leaning forward and sitting still. Low-pitched stridor with little or no cough.

Foreign Body

A foreign body may lead to a sudden onset of coughing and stridor with no fever.

Stridor

Assessment

Severe obstruction is indicated by:

(1) Marked stridor all the time.
(2) Child lies quiet and may be drowsy.
(3) The skin is pale and lips blue.
(4) There may be a distinct use of accessory muscles and inter-costal recession.

Do not examine the throat if there is any suspicion of acute epig-lottitis as this may precipitate respiratory and cardiac arrest.

105

Management

Admit—if there is any suspicion of epiglottitis; moderate or severe croup; or suspicion of foreign body.
Keep at home—if there is croup with mild stridor (treat with steam and amoxycillin (Amoxil); stay up with the child; and call again if condition worsens.

The child with asthma

Any lower respiratory tract infection may be associated with wheezing. Recurrent wheezy bronchitis is usually asthma and should be treated with bronchodilators rather than antibiotics.

A visit is advisable if the parents are worried by the child's breathing.

Assessment

The amount of audible wheezing is a poor indication of the severity of the bronchospasm. In severe bronchospasm the child lies still, is anxious and does not talk, is pale with blue lips, and there is inter-costal recession and use of accessory muscles. There is poor air entry—*beware* silent chest.

Management

One year and under (but is more likely due to bronchitis or bronchiolitis). Admit if bronchiolitis. If kept at home use steam, aminophylline suppositories 50 mg b.d., Phenergan elixir 5 ml b.d., amoxycillin.
Two years and over. Try 2 puffs of a ventolin or similar inhaler. Coordinate with inspiration if possible, but surprisingly effective even when this is not precise. If wheeze persists and is *mild to moderate* give salbutamol syrup 5 ml b.d. or t.d.s. *If severe* give sub-cutaneous terbutaline (Bricanyl):

    2 years 0.1 mg s.c.
    5 years 0.2 mg s.c.
    10 years 0.3 mg s.c.

and continuation treatment is oral salbutamol or aminophylline suppositories. If severe wheezing is not responding to treatment—*admit* and give i.v. hydrocortisone 100 mg before transfer.

The recurrent wheezer

Parents should keep a stock of suitable drugs at home. If known to have severe or persistent attacks may be give prednisolone to use in short courses.

The child who has fits

One child in twelve will have had a seizure of some sort by the age of 11 years. These are most likely to be febrile fits but if recurrent may be epilepsy.

The caller is usually very upset and is often afraid that the child is dying.

The risk of structural cause or subsequent epilepsy is greatest if: fit is prolonged; fits start below age of 1 year; it is a focal fit; or there are recurrent fits.

Telephone

Tell caller you will visit immediately and to put child into the recovery position and, if febrile, start tepid sponging.

Management

If fit stopped. Take careful history to establish whether it was a fit.

(1) If first fit admit to hospital
(2) In recurrent fits, if there is any suspicion that it may be meningitis—*admit*. Otherwise treat exactly as before, but keep at home; give tepid sponging; aspirin or paracetamol; rectal diazepam (Valium) 0.25 mg/kg (use a syringe without a needle).

If still having fit, i.v. diazepam (Valium) 0.125 mg/kg slowly. If you cannot get into a vein give rectal diazepam (Valium) 0.25 mg/kg. Then admit.

Follow-up

If the child is kept at home revisit after two hours. If there are recurrent fits consider need for prophylactic treatment.

The child with vomiting or diarrhoea or both

Vomiting and diarrhoea in a child may be associated with almost any physical or emotional illness. This is particularly true of vomiting. The younger the child the less specific are the symptoms. The importance of these symptoms is related entirely to the underlying cause and the extent of any associated dehydration.

Telephone

Make sure of what the caller means. Posseting or the normal loose stools of a baby may be regarded with alarm by inexperienced parents. The younger the child and the iller the child, the more important it is to see the child.

Assessment

Make a careful examination and history to determine the cause. In particular, check for otitis media, tonsillitis, meningitis or any abdominal disaster. Look for signs of dehydration: dry mouth, dry nappy, slack skin, depressed fontanelle and drowsy apathetic behaviour.

Management

Treatment, if any, should be for underlying cause. If gastroenteritis no antibiotics. If severe take a faecal sample for culture. For fluid replacement, give little and often—hourly if possible. Use water with three level teaspoons of glucose per 200 ml water, or diorylate (sodium chloride and dextrose oral powder compound), one sachet per 200 ml water, or lemonade or icecream soda for older children. *Do not* use salt or drinks with a lot of glucose.

Follow-up

Infants, if at all ill, must be revisited. Advise parents to call again if the child's condition deteriorates.

Abdominal pain in children

Most parents are worried about appendicitis when they call. This is likely to be uppermost in the doctor's mind as well. In virtually every instance the child must be seen, though if the history is short then a judicious delay may make diagnosis and assessment easier.

Assessment

Abdominal pain is often the presenting symptom of disease of other systems, so all systems need to be examined. Examine abdomen with great patience in the wriggling toddler, just keep your hand gently on the abdomen while the child is being cuddled on mother's lap.

Causes to remember

Evening colic in babies under 3 months. It is recurrent, the baby is well, parents anxious.
Colic due to gastroenteritis or respiratory tract infections.
Intussusception. Commonest at age 5–9 months. Severe colic but well in between spasms. Look for blood and take pulse rate.
Strangulated hernia or torsion of testes. Lower abdominal pain—diagnosis will be missed if child is not undressed.
Appendicitis. Often atypical in children—hence the need for obsessionally careful abdominal examination. If in doubt always re-examine later. It is dangerous to make a diagnosis of mesenteric adenitis.
Urinary tract infections. Urinary symptoms are often absent. High index of suspicion needed. Take mid-stream urine specimen.

Management

Treat underlying cause and admit if there is any suspicion of a surgical condition. Keep at home with clear instructions to call again if any worse. Revisit in ten hours if any cause for anxiety.

Emergencies in Adults

Abdominal Pain

Principles of management

Acute abdominal pain causes great anxiety in patients and relatives who always worry about appendicitis. Beware of bias, even in the most chronic of neurotics. They are just as likely to get an acute abdomen as anybody else.

Always see the patient—pain may sometimes be due to a severe disorder.

Assessment

A careful history will usually give you the diagnosis, but you will be caught out sooner or later if you do not perform a scrupulous examination including hernial orifices, bowel sounds and a rectal examination.

Appropriate disposal is more important than accurate diagnosis. The most important decision is: 'Is this an acute surgical condition?' Marked tenderness, guarding, rebound tenderness and constant pain all point to a surgical condition. Do not forget that in the early stages of obstruction the pain may be colicky with no physical signs in the abdomen.

Management

If acute surgical condition is suspected *admit*. If the condition is medical/cold surgical keep the patient under surveillance and try to reach a precise diagnosis. Refer as necessary.

Psychosocial Emergencies

Such emergencies are not very common but incidence does vary with practice area. They are disproportionately difficult to deal with. Formal diagnosis is not as important as the degree of disturbance that the patient is causing. Aberrant behaviour may be understandable in terms of reaction to events in the patient's life and is not a sign of mental illness.

The mental state of other involved people may be relevant—who is really the patient?

Resist being blackmailed into accepting responsibility for a problem unless you are convinced that the patient is unable to make logical decisions. Do not label a patient as 'mad' if there is any reasonable doubt.

Symptoms

Confusion

Patient is disorientated in time and place, but usually has lucid intervals, and is often restless and panicky. Hallucinations are possible. Condition is generally worse at night.

In the young. May be due to drugs or alcohol.
In the elderly it may be caused by cerebral arteriosclerosis with underlying illness.
Management. If drugs/alcohol are the cause arrange supervision by relatives. Look for and treat organic illness—e.g. heart failure. Resist demands to have elderly patient taken away as an emergency. Admission may make the patient worse, but is indicated if patient lives alone and is unmanageable. Bed in psychogeriatric unit or in Part III home often unavailable. Police have power to remove to a place of safety a patient found wandering.

Aggression/violence

Psychopaths who are often aggravated by drink, drugs, etc. Epilepsy or schizophrenia may be cause.

Police may be needed before, with, or instead of the doctor. Plan approach with police (no heroics).

If aggressive person is a psychopath better not to label patient as ill—he or she should take responsibility for consequences of behaviour.
If psychotic, patient may need admission under section 29.
If violence uncontrollable give 200 mg i.m. promazine (Sparine) while patient is restrained by others.

111

Acutely psychotic

Schizophrenia. Schizophrenic patients are usually young, often lapsed from treatment. May have delusions, which may be paranoid. Hallucinations, usually auditory. Behaviour may be bizzare.

Mania. Patient is excessively active in elated mood with no insight. Not usually violent unless restrained.

Depression. The patient may be guilt-ridden and retarded, some may be agitated. They cannot concentrate, have poor memory. There is a risk of suicide.

Management. If events out of control at home then arrange admission. Certify only if patient will not consent and if absolutely necessary. If agitated or excited give 200 mg i.m. promazine (Sparine).

Suicide threats/attempts

Hysterical. The patient is commonly a young woman who has taken tablets. She may be manipulative and action frequently follows family row/alcohol. Her attempt will have been well publicised.

Mentally ill. Generally among older patients. Methodical attempt. The attempt will not have been publicised.

Management. If *overdose* taken should be admitted to casualty. *Threat* from mentally ill must be taken seriously. Arrange psychiatric opinion/admission.

Threat from hysterical patient. Try to establish responsibility of patient for own actions and also responsibility of relatives and friends to supervise.

Anxiety/panic situational crisis

Neurosis. Usually a long standing neurotic. May be the result of family crisis. Relatives and patient tend to be demanding. Hyperventilation is common. This is not really a medical emergency—make this clear.

Management. Calm firm handling essential. Do not give in to demands and manipulation.

Bereavement/grief

Uninhibited expressions of normal emotion are often regarded as 'illness' in our culture. Callers expect doctor to give drugs to suppress feelings.

Management. Putting an arm round the shoulders or holding the hand of the bereaved person does more than drugs and teaches the relatives what is required. At the very most, give some diazepam (Valium) for one or two nights though a stiff gin and tonic would probably do just as well.

Compulsory admission of psychiatric patients

England and Wales

Compulsion must be used only if patient will not go voluntarily. Compulsion may be used when a patient suffers from a mental disorder that warrants detention in hospital when treament is necessary for the patient's health or for the safety of the patient or others.

DHSS recommend use of section 25 (observation) if at all possible but in most GP emergencies section 29 (emergency) is more practical.

Section 29, emergency. 72 hours. One medical recommendation is needed. One application signed by any relative or a social worker. Must state that using section 25 would cause unacceptable delay.

Section 25, observation. 28 days. Two medical recommendations necessary—one doctor with special psychiatric experience and one who has previous knowledge of the patient. One application by nearest relative or a social worker is needed. If the nearest relative objects social worker *cannot* apply.

Procedure. Medical recommendation precedes the application. Arrange application by social worker if possible because most relatives would rather not be involved. You must arrange a bed with the hospital—completing an order does not guarantee a bed.

(Always keep a Section 29 form in your bag, then you are not dependent on the social worker.)

Scotland

In emergency use Section 31 of Mental Health Act (Scotland) 1960.

One medical recommendation by doctor who has seen the patient that day necessary.

You must try to obtain consent of relative or mental officer: if not obtained you must state why. Patient can be detained for 7 days

Northern Ireland

In emergency use admission form 3 of Mental Health (Northern Ireland) Act 1961.

Part 1. Application by relative or social worker.
Part 2. Medical recommendation by doctor stating: when examined; clinical condition; why detention in hospital is needed and why informal admission is not suitable.

Patients can be detained for 7 days.

Acute Vertigo

Vertigo is a definite loss of spatial orientation—usually with a feeling of rotation—and most emergency calls are for a first attack.

Sudden onset of vertigo is frightening. Patients usually complain of being dizzy or giddy; make sure you find out exactly what the patient means.

Telephone

Acute vertigo, especially with vomiting, is distressing and, unless it is a recurrent problem, is a good reason for an emergency consultation.

Assessment

In an emergency the doctor's primary task is to exclude serious disease of the ear or central nervous system (CNS).

Ears. Check for any evidence of active middle-ear infection. Discharge from the middle ear means invasive infection until proved otherwise. Refer urgently.

If you can provoke vertigo with sudden pressure down the line of the external auditory meatus with the ball of your finger, this will confirm your diagnosis.

Occasionally wax or debris may be a cause. Check the hearing—sensorineural deafness may indicate a tumour or auditory neuroma.

Central Nervous System. Examine CNS carefully. Any CNS signs or symptoms would make you suspect a central vascular lesion, tumour or, in a young person, multiple sclerosis.

Eyes—nystagmus. Nystagmus has two components: slow deviation of eyes and rapid return to midline. The slow component is towards the side of the lesion. Signs of unilateral nystagmus are: lack of a latent period, non-fatiguability and nystagmus in any plane apart from the horizontal. These signs should make you suspect a central cause.

Central Nervous System. Check for evidence of cerebrovascular insufficiency—carotid bruits and vertebrobasilar artery syndrome.

Management

If patient still has vertigo when seen give prochlorperazine 25 mg (Stemetil) i.m., or as a suppository. When the acute attack is over, give oral prochlorperazine or similar drug, for a few days.

If there is middle-ear infection, or any possibility of serious CNS disease, refer urgently.

Follow-up

See patient 1–2 weeks later for review. If vertigo recurs, further evaluation will be necessary.

Eyes

Acutely painful and/or red eye

This is a common GP problem. If bilateral it is generally conjunctivitis. *Beware* the unilateral red/painful eye.

Loss of vision is possible from such conditions as herpetic keratitis or acute glaucoma. Careful evaluation: good lighting, loupe, sterile anaesthetic and fluorescein drops and an ophthalmoscope.

Telephone. See patient urgently if eye is definitely painful, rather than gritty, or if there is any loss of vision.

Assessment. See Table 14.7

Table 14.1 Eye assessment chart

Features	Acute conjunctivitis	Acute iritis	Acute glaucoma	Keratitis/corneal ulcer
Pain	Gritty rather than pain	Moderate Photophobia	Severe and radiating	Moderate
Discharge	Often pus	None	None	May occur
Visual disturbance	Smeared but no loss	Blurred	Gross with haloes	Blurred if area affected
Conjunctival injection	Peripheral	Around cornea	Diffuse	Around cornea or diffuse
Pupil/light reflex	Normal	Small, irregular, sluggish	Large, oval, fixed	Normal
Cornea	Clear	Clear or slightly hazy	Steamy	Ulcer or hazy patches
Intraocular pressure	Normal	Normal	High	Normal

Management
(1) *Acute iritis or keratitis*—urgent ophthalmic opinion required.
(2) *Acute glaucoma*—admit. Give buprenorphine (Temgesic) 0.3–0.6 mg i.m.
(3) *Large ulcer or dendritic ulcer, or herpes zoster*—refer for urgent ophthalmic opinion.
(4) *Small ulcer* on periphery or *minor abrasion*;
    (a) give cyclopentholate 0.5% 1–2 drops;
    (b) apply chloramphenicol ointment;
    (c) apply pad and bandage; review in 24 hours

Do not use steroid drops and *do not* pad conjunctivitis.

Arc eye

These are corneal flash burns due to ultraviolet light, usually caused by arc welding. Symptoms start several hours after exposure.

- Give amethocaine 1% and cyclopentholate 0.5% drops
- Pad and bandage
- Give oral analgesics.
- Review patient's condition in 48 hours.

Foreign bodies in eyes

Take a careful history to determine if there is any possibility of a penetrating injury, e.g. metal grinding or the use of hammer and chisel.

Assessment. Give amethocaine 1% drops to facilitate examination; fluorescein may be necessary to locate foreign body.
Management. If foreign body is large, deeply embedded or there is any possibility of a penetrating injury—send to ophthalmic casualty. Otherwise attempt removal with moist swab or the top of a hypodermic needle. If successful, apply chloromycetin ointment. Pad eye and review in 24 hours. If unsuccessful, refer patient to ophthalmic casualty department.

Sudden loss of vision

This is frightening and all patients need to be seen urgently. Unilateral loss or a field of defect may have been present for some time, but patient may only just have noticed it.

Assessment. First determine whether or not vision has actually been lost—try to eliminate hysterical loss of vision.

- *Is it longstanding?* It is not uncommon for a patient with slowly developing cataract to realise suddenly that there is unilateral loss of vision and then to panic.
- Look for—retinal artery occlusion—pale empty eyes;
  —retinal vein occlusion—congested with haemorrhages.
  —vitreous haemorrhage—blood obscures view of fundus.
  —retinal detachment—with field loss and dark bulge in retina.
- Consider the possibility of cranial arteritis or migraine.

Management. Any sudden and persistent loss of vision needs urgent referral. Often there is no remedy, but patient's anxiety needs relieving. Retinal detachment is most important because sight may be saved. Any small, sudden field loss, even if you cannot see a detachment on fundoscopy, needs *immediate* referral. Do not let the patient drive or undertake any exertion.

Alleged Assault

Telephone. Advise if casualty/police should be involved rather than you. if visit is necessary to record injuries rather than for treatment, arrange to see patient at your convenience.

Management. Make detailed record of injuries. If injuries are serious send to casualty. If minor, treat as necessary.

Alleged Indecent Assault or Rape

In these cases the police and a trained police surgeon ought to be involved. Strongly advise this from the onset. If you do see the patient then a lot of sympathy and tact is necessary. Do nothing which may confuse or destroy evidence.

Leave the gathering of evidence to a police surgeon unless you are suitably trained yourself.

What to do with a Dead Body

Whether or not a death is expected it is reasonable and kind to visit to confirm death, give moral support and advice to relatives, and make sure about the circumstances of death.

Assessment.

Diagnosis of death. Be careful, you will look silly if the patient wakes up later in the mortuary. Look for:

- absent pulse
- absent heart sounds
- absent corneal and pupillary reflexes
- engorged retinal vessels.

If circumstances are suspicious—look for:

- injuries
- strange attitudes or situation
- possibility of a poison.

Can you issue a certificate?

Yes—if you are satisfied death is natural and patient has been seen during the last 14 days
No—If patient not seen during the last 14 days, if cause is unknown, if violent or accidental, or if connected with operation of anaesthetic.

The coroner must also be informed when death is (1) from industrial disease, (2) in a patient with a pensioned disability, (3) suicide, (4) poisoning or due to drugs, (5) due to want, exposure or neglect, or (6) if any criticism of medical or nursing care is likely.

Management

Expected natural death. Confirm death and tell family to contact undertaker if this is desired. If only elderly or distressed spouse in house, you could do this.

Arrange for death certificate to be issued when convenient. Ask if cremation is intended and, if so, arrange for second medical certificate. If pacemaker is *in situ*—warn undertaker.

119

Unexpected death or if not seen in last 14 days. Confirm death and inform duty officer at police station. Give full details and your assessment of the situation. Do not allow the body to be removed.

If you are **reasona**bly certain death was due to natural causes, the coroner **may give** you permission to issue an endorsed certificate (initialled in box A on reverse of form).

15. BREAD AND BUTTER PROBLEMS

Managing apparently minor disorders accounts for a large proportion of the GP's basic workload. As most of these conditions are hardly seen in hospital, or taught at medical school, trainees may initially experience difficulties in dealing with them. The brief notes which follow are designed to provide you with enough helpful, albeit dogmatic, information to allow you to cope satisfactorily until discussion with your trainer and further reading determine your individual views and management patterns.

Remember that although most of these conditions are trivial in a purely medical sense, they can provoke disproportionate anxiety and worry. Careful explanation is a vital part of management. Where explanation appears not to be readily accepted it is worth trying to discover what the patient feels or fears about the condition. Unless anxieties are ventilated and then allayed the consultation will not have a satisfactory outcome.

Acne

Occurs as a reaction to sex hormone changes and affects four out of five teenagers. Blackheads and pimples on the face, back and chest look unsightly but in most cases they will clear up in the late teens or early 20s.

Frequent washing with soap and water and getting as much sunlight as possible will help; changing the diet will not and neither will squeezing the spots.

Anti-acne lotions or creams can be bought at the chemists or a cheap benzylperoxide preparation prescribed. Severe cases may be helped by a 3-month course of oxytetracycline 250 mg twice a day.

NB No tetracycline if there is any risk of pregnancy.

Allergic rashes

May be either a local contact dermatitis or a more generalised urticaria. Whatever the rash looks like it is likely to be sudden in onset and itchy. Urticaria may spread over large areas of the skin and may cause swelling (puffy eyes/difficulty in breathing). It generally clears up after a few days.

Identifying the cause and avoiding it may not be as easy as it sounds. An antihistamine may be prescribed for a few days if symptoms justify it.

NB Contrary to popular belief an allergy can develop only to an allergen that the body has previously become sensitised to.

Amenorrhoea

Best assumed to be caused by pregnancy until proved otherwise. Associated frequency, nausea or vomiting, faintness, breast soreness or tingling, sleepiness and constipation confirm the diagnosis without any need for pregnancy tests.

NB Anxiety and emotional upset may well cause amenorrhoea and so may thyrotoxicosis.

Athlete's foot

A fungal infection by no means confined to athletes. It starts between the toes, especially the little ones, with irritation and peeling of the skin which may spread to include the sole.

Keeping the feet clean and dry and avoiding tight-fitting footwear will help. Antifungal creams and powders may be prescribed or bought cheaply at the chemist and should be used regularly not just until irritation abates but until the skin between the toes returns completely to normal.

NB Shoe dermatitis will not respond to fungicides.

Balanitis

Presents with soreness, redness of the foreskin or glans and—often profuse—discharge. It should not be confused with a red ammoniacal foreskin from nappy rash or with paraphimosis. If it occurs in older males than venereal disease, diabetes and carcinoma of the penis should be excluded.

Any antiseptic cream may be used locally and, if infection looks severe, a penicillin may be prescribed. Recurrent infection associated with phimosis may necessitate circumcision.

NB The foreskin does not usually retract until a child is 2–3 years old.

Baldness

Male pattern, which starts in the late teens and slowly progresses, is so common as not to be abnormal.

In women the hair thins mainly on the top of the head and total loss will not occur. Thinning may be caused by tight plaits or sleeping in rollers or, rarely, by anaemia or myxoedema. Temporary loss may follow pregnancy, stopping the pill or an illness with a high fever.

When there is fairly sudden onset of patchy loss (alopecia) the hair will, in most cases, regrow within 2–3 months though the larger the bald area the less likely it is that regrowth will be complete.

NB Although there are no scalp preparations that will affect the outcome human nature being what it is many are likely to be tried.

Bell's palsy

Refers to an isolated benign unilateral paralysis of the facial nerve. Onset is rapid and often accompanied by a dull ache or wooden feeling round the ear. The affected side of the face may seen to have lost its expression and on smiling is drawn across to the unaffected side. Often the eyes cannot close completely. Sensory testing is normal. In severer cases there may be hyperacusis and loss of taste. In the absence of other symptoms indicating a more widespread neurological disease, oroscopic examination to exclude chronic middle-ear disease is all that is necessary.

With partial paralysis recovery will begin in 7–10 days and be complete in about 6 weeks. With total paralysis most people recover completely but a minority will not, though they may improve after 3 months or so. Simple analgesics, strict oral hygiene, taping the eyelid down at night, and regular gentle massaging of the affected muscles may help as may early high dose corticosteroid therapy (20 mg three times a day reducing by 5 mg daily).

NB In rare bilateral cases check the urine for sugar.

Birth marks

May be *portwine stains*, which are present at birth as red, slightly raised areas; they do not spread further but persist throughout life without any improvement, or *strawberry naevi* which appear within the first week of life as a small red spot then rapidly enlarge, to become deep red and raised above the skin surface, until the age of 18 months after which they remain static until the age of 3 years when they start to shrink to disappear completely by 5–6 years.

There is no real treatment in either case though portwine stains especially can be cosmetically camouflaged with covering creams.

NB careful sympathetic explanation of the natural history is essential.

Blepharitis

In its common form blepharitis is an outpost of dandruff from the scalp affecting the lid margins so that they become red, crusted and itchy. For effective treatment the dandruff must be controlled; crusts and discharge removed by cotton wool and water; and an antibiotic ointment (chloramphemical) applied three times a day.

NB Recurrence is highly likely.

Boils

These start around a hair root then spread into the surrounding skin. They are usually single but may be multiple or recurrent.

Dry heat may be used to help pointing, when incision and drainage will be more effective in producing resolution than antibiotics. Incision of large boils may require a general anaesthetic.

NB Recurrent boils may be due to diabetes but are more likely to be due to reinfection by staphylococci from the nares, genitalia or axillae.

123

Bunions

Typically develop in middle-aged women as the big toe is pushed permanently outwards, probably by ill-fitting shoes, and a bursa develops over the medial aspect of the first metatarsophalangeal joint.

A chiropodist may be able to help but surgical treatment is likely to be necessary in severe, painful cases.

NB Infection of the overlying bursa is not uncommon.

Carpal tunnel syndrome

Mostly occurs in overweight, middle-aged housewives who, by constant flexing and extending of the wrist, damage the median nerve within the carpal tunnel. A minority of cases arise as a feature of an underlying disease—e.g. old fracture, acromegaly, myxoedema, oedema (especially in pregnancy when it will resolve after delivery).

Pain—which may radiate up the arm—tingling and numbness are felt in the hand and fingers in the median nerve distribution. Attacks are most common at night, often waking the patient, and are relieved by shaking the hand or hanging the affected arm out of the bed.

Cases with severe or recurrent symptoms or any objective signs of neurological deficit in the hands must be treated with early surgical decompression. For milder symptoms relief may be gained by resting the hand and wrist (a resting night splint helps); a short course of a non-steroidal anti-inflammatory drug; weight reduction; and a diuretic if symptoms are worse premenstrually or aggravated by oedema from other causes.

NB The adductor pollicis is the only thenar eminence muscle spared.

Catarrh

Normally means a more than usual amount of secretions coming from the nose or bronchi. It may result from an oversensitive mucosa reacting to irritants, including dust and pollen, or infection. Thick yellow or green nasal discharge is usual.

In the absence of a treatable cause antibiotics are unlikely to give anything other than temporary relief as are nasal decongestant drops.

NB First find out what the patient means by catarrh.

Chickenpox

Highly infectious, usually mild, illness with an incubation period of 15–18 days and period of infectivity from one day before to 6 days after the rash. The rash is usually the first sign of infection and the vesicles come in crops, crusting within 7 days of arising.

If there is no chest, ear or sinus infection then treatment is purely symptomatic. Calamine lotion may be applied to itchy spots.

NB One attack confers lifelong immunity.

Colds

Common and usually self-treated. If patients come to the doctor it may be for a sick note; examination to exclude complications (babies are often brought because of worries that the cold has 'gone to the chest'); or in the hope or expectation of a prescription.

Unless sinusitis, bronchitis or otitis media are present no prescription is necessary though babies may benfit from nasal drops (ephedrine 0.5% 15 minutes before feeds) and chronic bronchitics etc from early antibiotics. General advice about symptomatic treatment should be given to everyone.

NB Non-prescribing for simple self-limiting conditions encourages patients to treat themselves the next time.

Cold sores

Caused by the herpes simplex virus which lies dormant in the skin repeatedly flaring up to produce, usually at the same site, painful sores on the lips, nose or cheeks.

Healing normally occurs within 10 days though surgical spirit or toilet water applied 3–4 hourly may speed this up. Ice applied to the sores has also been reported to be effective.

NB If severe and recurrent, idoxuridine (Herpid) used as soon as symptoms begin may be effective though likely effect must be balanced against expense.

Colic (3 months or evening)

Attacks usually begin within the first 15 days of life and recur nightly until at from 10–16 weeks they resolve completely. During attacks the baby's face becomes red, he draws his legs up, emits piercing screams and cannot be comforted. After 2–20 minutes pain suddenly ceases though regular recurrences last until about 10–11 at night when sleep supervenes.

Gentle pressure or massage of the abdomen, placing baby on his tummy and giving a breast or bottle to suck may all give some relief during an attack. Dicyclomine hydrochloride (Merbentyl) syrup 5 mg in 5 ml 15 minutes before feeds may also help.

NB Reassurance and explanation go a long way to helping the mother to cope.

Conjunctivitis

The commonest cause of red eyes and this condition is characterised by generalised conjunctival infection; discharge, most noticeable on waking; grittiness, rather than pain; and, if present, very mild photophobia. Visual acuity is unchanged and the pupil is normal.

Antibiotic drops (chloramphenicol) used 2–3 hourly, or more frequently if necessary, should be prescribed and the discharge kept clear with cotton wool and water. The eye should not be padded.

NB Unilateral conjunctivitis should not be diagnosed so readily as bilateral conjunctivitis.

Cradle cap

Tends to appear first at about 1 month of age and clears up at 6 months. The yellow brown greasy scalp scaling is very common and usually mild though occasionally it may be severe with thick yellow lumps rather than scales.

A mild keratolytic, e.g. cetrimide (Cetavlex) cream should be applied at night and shampooed out the next morning with a simple shampoo.

NB Hair growth will not be affected in any way.

Dandruff

If dry, white, scaly and present for long periods, may be the only evidence of a seborrhoeic tendency. Severe scalp scaling may also be caused by psoriasis (patchy with palpable lesions) or atopic eczema and ichthyosis (past history and evidence of flexural lesions elsewhere on body).

Mild cases respond to detergent shampoos while severer dry scaling will be helped by selenium sulphide (Lenium, Selsun). These shampoos should be advised but not prescribed, though for psoriatic or eczematous scalps Polytar shampoo or Betnovate scalp application may be.

Dysmenorrhoea

Most often affects young women and may start a day or two before the bleeding. Malaise, headache, nausea may also occur and there may be a link with constipation. It is not a sign of disease but if it is severe or a new symptom a vaginal examination should be carried out.

Sufferers should be advised to continue with all normal physical activities; avoid constipation at period time; and to try to resolve any contributory emotional problems. Soluble aspirin is a useful analgesic though if pain is still severe a non-steroidal anti-inflammatory agent may be prescribed.

NB This is one condition greatly relieved by the pill.

Earache

Associated with an upper respiratory infection and a red drum is caused by otitis media. A normal drum but tender pinna would suggest an external meatal boil while intermittent pain with a normal ear suggests a dental origin. Hard wax may be the cause but it is wise to check the drum after syringing.

In all cases simple analgesics should be advised. Dry heat may help a boil to point while antibiotics are necessary in most, but certainly not all, cases of otitis media. Penicillin V is the antibiotic of choice except in 1–5 year olds when amoxycillin (Amoxil) is favoured.

NB Babies cannot complain of earache and so rely on you to make the diagnosis for them.

Eczema

Caused by primary irritants and allergy, eczema may be easily diagnosed on the basis of the distribution of the rash and an adequate history (including occupation and hobbies). Prevention of further exposure of the skin to the substance responsible for the reaction is of paramount importance. One per cent hydrocortisone cream applied 3 or 4 times a day will help though sometimes a more potent preparation may be needed.

Atopic eczema affects about 10% of children and in the vast majority it will clear permanently in childhood. It is usually mild and begins after the age of 3 months, most often affecting flexures then face, neck and hands. Parents must be warned that exacerbations are characteristic and that creams like 1% hydrocortisone are suppressive not curative. Stronger steroids should be used only in short courses if the eczema proves refractory.

NB This is not a contraindication to any vaccination except smallpox.

Enuresis

Not a disease, but delayed development of bladder control. At 3 years 75% of children are dry by night; at 6 years 92%; and at 12 years virtually all. In less than 3% of primary enuretics there will be an underlying organic abnormality, e.g. mental retardation, lesion of the lower spinal cord, urinary tract abnormalities. Secondary enuresis developing after the child has achieved control may be due to the onset of urinary infection, diabetes or epilepsy but it is far more likely to be caused by a sudden emotional disturbance.

After the age of 5–6 treatment may be justified. Parents should be advised *to praise and reward* for dry nights; empty bladder before bed; lift as late as possible and be first one up in morning, and *not* to scold, blackmail or threaten, comment or tease about wet nights, restrict fluid intake, or increase salt in food. A chart of wet/dry nights allows the true frequency of wetting to be assessed, imipramine 25 mg at night will help high frequency wetters within a week and may reduce family tensions but has a high relapse rate; a pad and buzzer alarm will produce a long-term cure in 80% of cases.

NB Urinalysis and mid-stream urine specimen should be examined on presentation and if there is any recurrence.

Epistaxis

This comes predominantly from local trauma-related causes. Most cases are dealt with at home using simple first aid. Active bleeding should be treated with even and firm pressure applied to the anterior nasal septum by pinching the nostrils closed between thumb and forefinger. While the patient mouth breathes pressure is maintained for at least 5 minutes. Careful examination of the nose (using an auriscope) is best carried out when no bleeding is taking place.

Mild recurrent bleeds associated with nasal crusting may be helped by topical use of soft paraffin three times a day to soften the discharge, and localised nasal infection may be treated by an antibiotic cream. Frequent recurrences may need ENT referral for cautery to Little's area.

NB Severe or recurrent bleeding warrants a full blood count.

Flat feet

Normal when a child starts to stand because the medial arch does not develop until the second or third year of life. After this age if the feet are still flat but are painfree with normal mobility and muscle power no treatment is necessary, though insoles may help shoe wear.

Feet that are painful, stiff or hypermobile, and weak or spastic may be part of a generalised condition, e.g. cerebral palsy, or indicate a local bony or inflammatory problem that needs diagnosis and treatment.

NB Getting a child to stand on tiptoe will accentuate the medial arch.

Fleas

Fleas generally drop off domestic pets onto furniture and carpets. A typical bite is urticarial with a central punctum and surrounding flare and may develop into quite a large blister. Bites tend to occur on exposed areas (below the knee, arms, hands) and discrete papules may persist for some months.

Furniture and carpets should be treated with an insecticide containing pyrethrum; pets should be treated by the vet; and antihistamines may be prescribed to relieve irritation.

NB Persisting papules are often not suspected of being flea bites.

Foreign body in the ear

Rarely causes damage comparable to that caused by ill-advised attempts at extraction. Some foreign bodies, e.g. paper, may be easily removed by syringing or blunt forceps but if the patient is not likely to be cooperative and quite still and if the doctor is not experienced in using a blunt right-angled probe (passed beyond foreign body and gently withdrawn) and head mirror then referral to casualty or ENT is indicated.

NB Filling the ear with water will kill a live insect and give much relief.

Foreign body in the eye

Demands a careful history to exclude any possibility of a penetrating injury—e.g. from metal grinding, use of hammer and chisel. If penetration was possible, the eye injured, or the foreign body deeply embedded in the cornea then the patient should be referred direct to casualty. If none of the problems are present 1% amethocaine drops should be used for pain relief to allow careful eye examination (including subtarsal area). The foreign body may be removed with a moist cotton wool swab or, if practised, an embedded particle may be removed using a hypodermic needle.

Once removed, the eye should be stained with fluorescein to assess damage, chloramphenicol drops instilled, eye padded for 12 hours, and the patient seen again in 48 hours to recheck the cornea.

NB If there is any possibility of penetration – even if the patient feels only vaguely that something is in the eye—this is an ocular emergency.

Foreign body in the nose

If not removed by forcible nose blowing and not easily seen and grasped by forceps or got behind by angled probe then refer direct to ENT. Definite risk of inhalation so immediate referral necessary.

NB Consider this in any child with foul-smelling unilateral discharge.

Glandular fever

Generally affects teenagers and though not very infectious may develop 1–2 weeks after contact with a case. Most patients feel ill with a swinging temperature and a very sore throat which may persist for weeks associated with lymphadenopathy. A rash or jaundice may develop and while children tend to recover quickly adults may feel below par for weeks after an attack.

A Monospot test will confirm the diagnosis. No treatment, other than plenty of fluids and regular simple analgesics, will have any effect.

NB Suspect this in any teenager with a severe sore throat not responding to penicillin.

Halitosis

Tends to be a temporary state that will resolve naturally. If persistent it is likely to be the result of personal habits—e.g. stale tobacco smoke, spicy, garlic-laden foods, alcohol, poor dental care. It is seldom caused by any serious disease though it may be associated with chronic nasal and chest infections.

Advice may be given on personal habits or a visit to the dentist suggested. If ENT examination reveals purulent postnasal or nasal discharge an antibiotic might be prescribed.

NB Most smells come from anaerobic bacteria so metronidazole (Flagyl) might well be the antibiotic of choice.

Hay fever

A grass-pollen allergy causing coryza-like symptoms, conjunctival irritation and even wheezing in sensitive individuals seasonally from late May to mid-July. A common problem, it usually begins in the teens and recurs annually for 5–15 years until natural resolution occurs. Diagnosis presents few problems—but non-grass pollen allergies are less dramatic in their presentation and occur at different times of the year—and is simply based on history.

Symptom severity is proportional to atmospheric pollen count and sufferers should avoid walking through long grass, camping, car or train journeys with open windows, and house windows open on hot, humid, windy days though complete avoidance of pollen is impractical. Other than these measures, mild symptoms need no treatment beyond the wearing of sunglasses and the liberal use of hankies.

Social factors—e.g. type of employment, driving, important forthcoming events—are as important as the severity of symptoms in deciding treatment. Vasoconstrictor nose drops are useful in an emergency; antihistamines may need to be changed around to find the one most suitable for a particular patient or when tolerance develops; topical disodium cromoglycate and steroids are costly and not always well tolerated; systemic steroids may be justified for severe symptoms or to tide the patient over an important event; desensitisation courses, if indicated, should be completed at least three weeks before the expected start of the season.

NB It is well worth taking time initially to explain the aetiology of the condition and self-help measures available.

Hyperhidrosis

In hot humid weather hyperhidrosis may produce the itchy rash of prickly heat, though when patients complain of excess perspiration they are usually referring to local sweating. Very sweaty feet macerate the skin and give an unpleasant smell. Very sweaty axillae and palms are usually caused by emotional tension and typically affect female teenagers.

Feet can be helped by avoiding rubber-soled shoes, wearing sandals wherever possible and soaking the soles of the feet in 3% formalin solution for 5–10 minutes each night. Prickly heat is helped by wearing little and loose clothing, using fans to cool the skin surface and limiting activity to reduce sweating. Axillary sweating is helped by wearing sleeveless dresses, not overusing underarm deodorants and trying to reduce tension and stress. In severe cases application of a 20% solution of aluminium chloride hexahydrate in absolute alcohol painted on nightly for one week is effective though hydrocortisone ointment may be needed for irritant skin reaction. Excision of apocrine gland areas may be necessary.

NB Heat-induced sweating is normal and requires no treatment.

Impetigo

An epidermal infection by *Staphylococcus aureus* or a streptococcus. Superficial spreading yellow crusts are usually found on the face and hands. Circinate lesions with less distinct crusting and a clearly defined spreading edge may occur. Satellite lesions are common.

Careful personal hygiene is necessary to stop the spread and a topical antibiotic, e.g. sodium fusidate (Fucidin) should be used four times a day until all signs of the disorder are cleared. A course of penicillin may be given if the condition is extensive or recurrent.

NB Many schools insist on keeping children away until their impetigo has completely cleared up. This is unnecessary and may be avoided if the doctor confines his diagnosis to 'a skin infection'.

Influenza

Term used by both doctors and patients for feverish upper respiratory tract infections seldom due to any specific virus. Malaise, fever, cough, coryza, aching and sweating last 2–3 days and are followed by gradual improvement. Most cases are uncomplicated and benign but in epidemic influenza there is a case fatality rate of 1 in 500 (mainly in the elderly).

General measures are all that is necessary unless secondary bacterial infection supervenes. Antibiotics should be used sooner rather than later in the elderly and patients with chronic cardiac or respiratory conditions.

NB Malaria cases are often wrongly diagnosed as flu.

Ingrowing toenails

Mainly confined to the big toenails of teenage boys. Medical advice is usually sought when infection develops in the skin round the nail.

Mild infections can be treated by antibiotic creams while more severe infections will need an oral antibiotic. Good foot hygiene, going barefoot or in sandals wherever possible, and cutting the toenail at a right angle to the long axis of the toe may help. Cutting away the ingrowing part of the nail may be necessary.

Severe or persistent cases may require surgical referral for removal of the nail.

NB Your trainer may have his own minor operation for dealing with this problem.

Insect bites and stings

Mainly from bees and wasps, will present because of pain, swelling or fears of local infection. A bee sting can be scraped out with a finger nail and the site should be cleaned with antiseptic. Soluble aspirin is an effective analgesic and unless swelling is marked and spreading—when an antihistamine may be prescribed—or secondary infection appears to be present—when an antibiotic may be needed—the patient should be advised that symptoms will resolve within 2–3 days.

NB A few people are hypersensitive to bee or wasp venom and may be killed by a single sting.

Insomnia

Not a disease *per se* but it may be a symptom of physical or psychological disorder. Most often it is a normal sleep pattern variation which for some reason has become unacceptable.

Any underlying disease should be treated in its own right—e.g. depression with antidepressants; pain with analgesics. When there is no underlying disease, explanation that sleep needs differ from person to person and from time to time and will sort themselves out should be given. It is worth saying that an elderly person averages only 4–5 hours sleep a night and that catnapping during the day is just as good as sleep at night. Simple advice on improving sleep quality can be given, namely, a regular routine at night with a walk or hot bath, hot milky drink and a quiet book; no television or work in the bedroom; comfortable bed and surroundings.

If prescribed at all, hypnotics should be prescribed for only a short course and it should be made clear to the patient that when the tablets are finished no more will be forthcoming.

NB The best way to avoid hypnotic dependence is by not prescribing in the first place.

Intoeing

Where the toes turn in, or one leg is thrown around the other, or the child falls over his own feet, is fairly common when walking begins. In most cases the cause lies above the knee so that the foot is normal and the child walks with the whole leg turned in and the knees facing a little towards each other. This nearly always corrects itself by the age of 6 and only if it is still severe then or appears for the first time after then would an orthopaedic opinion be needed.

Metatarsus varus, where the forefoot turns inward relative to the hindfoot, is usually recognised before the child starts to walk. Eight out of nine cases will correct themselves without treatment by the age of 3. Severe or persistent cases may need an orthopaedic opinion.

NB Waiting to make sure the abnormality will not correct by itself does not make it any more difficult to treat later.

Knock knees

Symmetrically present, to some degree, in 75% of 2–4$\frac{1}{2}$ year olds. In 99 cases out of 100 this is a normal variation and will correct itself without treatment by the age of 7 years.

Pronounced asymmetry, short stature, an intermalleolar separation (measured with the child lying down) of $3\frac{1}{2}$ in or condition uncorrected by 10–11 years would warrant orthopaedic opinion.

NB No damage will be caused by waiting for a child to grow out of mild knock knees and seeking further opinion only if it does not.

Laryngitis

This condition, with hoarse cough and hoarse or lost voice, is easily diagnosed. Symptoms may be part of a viral upper respiratory tract infection in which case general measures, including resting the voice, are all that is necessary and most patiently will recover fully within 3–7 days. If there is evidence of sinusitis or severe systemic upset a broad spectrum antibiotic should be prescribed.

NB Any hoarseness persisting for more than three weeks demands urgent ENT referral for laryngoscopy.

Lice

Seen mostly in children's heads, where the main symptom is itching.

They are contagious and the eggs laid close to the scalp become attached to growing hairs and develop into nits (small white specks firmly attached to the hair shafts). All members of the family should be treated at the same time by washing the hair, then applying malathion 0.5% solution liberally, leaving for 12 hours, then shampooing the scalp again and combing the wet hair with a fine-tooth comb. Treatment is best repeated in one week.

Pubic lice are treated in the same way (without fine-tooth combing) but if found the question of whether other venereal diseases are present or not should be raised.

NB Nits cannot be brushed off, whereas dandruff can.

Lumps and bumps

Those proffered for an opinion include lipomas, lymph nodes, papillomas, sebaceous cysts, ganglia, warts, moles, boils, rodent ulcers and so on. Presentation is either for reassurance that nothing serious is amiss or for removal of the offending lump on cosmetic or other grounds.

If the patient wishes it, or if there is any suspicion whatsoever of malignancy, removal should be arranged either within the practice or at a hospital outpatient clinic.

NB Multiple lipomas may be neurofibromas.

Measles

Highly infectious with an incubation period of 10–14 days followed by 3–4 days of feverish upper respiratory tract infection symptoms before the development of the characteristic maculopapular rash. Pyrexia may persist for the first 2–3 days of the rash after which the child's conditions rapidly improves. The infectious stage lasts for 5 days before the rash appears to 5 days after the temperature is back to normal.

Acute otitis media and chest infection are the main complications requiring antibiotic treatment. Management otherwise is on general lines with plenty of fluids, 4-hourly paracetamol, bed rest if the child desires it, and possibly an antihistamine cough medicine—e.g. Phenergan (promethazine Hcl), at night for its sedative effect.

NB During a measles epidemic it is wise to say to all parents that their child's cold may be prodromal measles.

Meibomian cyst

Granuloma occurring in a Meibomian gland giving rise to a chronic painless (unless infection develops) swelling usually situated at some distance from the lid margin. Eyes referral is required for incision and curettage as spontaneous resolution will not occur.

NB Pain implies abscess formation.

Menopause

Retrospectively diagnosed occurs on average at age 51 when women may already be experiencing anxieties about future functioning, doubts about their attractiveness and sexuality, and fears of approaching old age. Sudden hormone changes may be associated with unpleasant symptoms, many of which are coincidental and as likely to be helped by placebo as oestrogen. Symptoms of vasomotor instability (flushes, sweats and flush-induced insomnia) and of urogenital atrophy may be oestrogen-deficiency related. Only a minority of women will feel that their menopausal symptoms warrant a medical opinion.

A sympathetic ear in itself may be therapeutic and avoidance of stress and alcohol will decrease flushing. Atrophic vaginitis may be helped by using KY jelly for lubrication during intercourse or by oestrogen-containing creams. Vasomotor symptoms if severe may be temporarily allayed by minor tranquillisers, clonidine, Bellergal (a mixture of phenobarbitone and belladonna) or ethinyloestradiol 10 micrograms three times a day for 2–3 months. There are many arguments against long-term hormone replacement therapy which are beyond the scope of this book.

NB Contraception should be used for 2 years after the presumed last period if the woman is below 50 and for one year if she is over 50.

Moles

Moles, or pigmented naevi, are not all present at birth and may appear in childhood. Every adult has some—on average 15–20. Their importance lies in the very small chance they have of developing into malignant melanomata. Sudden enlargement, alteration in pigmentation of the lesion or the surrounding skin, and bleeding or ulceration of the lesion should all raise the suspicion of malignancy.

Other reasons for surgical excision are cosmetic and where the lesion is prominently situated on part of the skin which is subject to trauma from clothing.

NB No other forms of treatment should be attempted.

Mouth ulcers

Usually multiple, sore, and shallow, about 2–10 mm in diameter and found on the tongue, floor of the mouth and inside of the cheeks. These aphthous ulcers each take about 4–10 days to heal and the tendency to develop them persists for many years. No treatment is effective, but avoiding smoking, hot food and ill-fitting dentures may help as may good dental hygiene.

Single persistent ulcers may be from a rough tooth or denture though the possibility of malignancy should be considered.

NB Soluble aspirin gargled then swallowed is as helpful as anything else.

Mumps

Essentially a benign disease and even in complicated cases (orchitis, oophoritis, pancreatitis, aseptic meningitis), complete recovery with no sequelae is the rule. Incubation period is 18–21 days with the patient being infectious for 2–3 days before the swelling occurs and remaining so until the glands have returned to normal size.

Mild constitutional upset may be experienced for a day or two before and after salivary gland (mainly parotid) enlargement appears. Swelling is often better seen than felt and characteristically one parotid pushes the earlobe upward and forwards while obliterating the groove between the ramus of the jaws and the mastoid process.

Children are little affected and need no more than simple analgesics and a good fluid intake. Adults may feel the need for bed rest.

Orchitis symptoms can be dramatically relieved by a short course of prednisolone (15 mg four times a day for four days).

NB Although children with mumps should be kept away from adults there is a strong case for trying to ensure that other children catch the infection.

Nappy rash

Primary irritation of the skin by prolonged contact with wet or dirty nappies, aggravated by the moisture-retaining action of plastic pants, characteristically spares the skin creases and folds. The inflamed and broken skin easily becomes secondarily infected with candida (isolated spots in the nappy area or failure to respond to simple measures suggests this) or pyogenic bacteria. Spread into the creases or out of the nappy area may occur in an atopic baby as a smoother, more shiny rash than usual or as napkin psoriasis.

Nappies should be changed as soon as possible after they become wet or soiled. The baby's bottom should be washed and thoroughly dried before being left exposed for as long as possible before a new nappy, with liner, is put on. Plastic pants should be avoided until the rash clears. In mild cases a simple emollient ointment such as zinc and castor oil may be used but where secondary infection is suspected an ointment like Nystaform HC (contains nystatin, clioquinol and hydrocortisone) should be used three times a day. Oral or maternal thrush should be treated at the same time.

NB Mother must understand that her care of the baby is the single most important factor in effecting a cure.

Nasal polyps

Follow either prolonged allergic rhinitis or chronic sinusitis and present with nasal obstruction, mouth breathing, snoring and loss of sense of smell. The polyp is a round, shiny grey obstruction which can be seen filling the nasal passage.

Treatment is surgical but recurrence after removal is likely.

NB Mechanical obstruction is unlikely to be helped by any medication.

Night cramps

Precipitated by random muscle contraction or voluntary stretching movements are quite a common cause of sleep disturbance in the elderly.

Keeping the bedclothes loose may help as may quinine sulphate 300 mg at night. Nevertheless, stretching exercises (stand three feet from wall, heels on floor, control forward tilt by hands outstretched onto wall. Stretch until moderate pulling sensation experienced in calves for 10 seconds then come back to upright posture to relax for 10 seconds before repeating. Continue for 5–10 minutes three times a day until cured) will cure most cases within a month or two.

NB Although explaining the exercises may initially take longer than prescribing, the time and money saved by not having to prescribe repeatedly more than compensates.

Obesity

A topic about which several books have been written. For practical purposes it is sufficient to say that group therapy (Weight Watchers, etc) is far more likely to achieve sustained weight reduction than the GP. It is worth giving enthusiasts a diet sheet and offering to reweigh them in 1–2 weeks but the importunings of 'yoyo' fatties for prescriptions for diuretics or appetite suppressants should be firmly resisted.

NB A well-trained practice nurse can deal with the practice's dieters as well as any doctor.

Otitis externa

Presents with itching or irritation, discharge and, possibly, pain in the ears. It is usually a recurrent problem which will flare up if the external canal becomes wet.

Treatment with a combination antibacterial/steroid drops—e.g. Locorten-vioform four times a day—will often be all that is needed. If infection is severe an oral broad-spectrum antibiotic should also be given.

NB If infection persists despite treatment check the urine for sugar.

Out-toeing

Charlie Chaplin-like walk is quite common within the first 2 years of life. It may be more pronounced on one side than the other and although most cases correct spontaneously with time it is important to make sure that the hips and spine are normal.

NB This may make the child appear to have very flat feet.

Piles

May present with fresh bleeding at the end of defecation, prolapse, irritation and itching, and pain. If untreated, spontaneous improvement will occur but recurrence is likely particularly if constipation is not avoided. However strong a past history the GP should not be deterred from performing a rectal examination in any adult with symptoms of piles to try to exclude carcinoma of rectum. If there is any suspicion of bowel cancer, sigmoidoscopy should be arranged.

Simple suppositories or creams such as Anusol or Anusol HC will help soothe the pain and discomfort. A high-fibre diet will help avoid constipation and good anal hygiene will help decrease irritation. Recurrent problems may justify injection or haemorrhoidectomy.

NB Creams containing local anaesthetics may ease anal pain initially but as they act as potent sensitisers may cause more irritation in the end.

Pityriasis rosea

Usually begins with the solitary herald patch. This is on the trunk and is a reddish brown annular scaly patch. Within 1–2 weeks other lesions appear on the trunk and tend to remain confined to the vest and pants area. These lesions may be oval macules, with their long axes in the lines of cleavage of the skin, or pink papules.

Apart from occasional irritation the disease is symptomless and will clear within 2–3 months of onset.

NB Once the patient has been assured of the benign self-limiting nature of the disease no active treatment is necessary.

Premenstrual syndrome

Refers to a wide range of psychic and somatic symptoms occurring in the 10–14 days before menstruation, and resolving for at least 7 days after. Those most often described are irritability, depression, exhaustion, panic, painful or tender breasts, oedema, stomach ache, nausea and headache. The basic cause is unknown though psychological factors play a part and it seems fair to assume some direct or indirect hormone influences are at work.

Sympathetic, clear explanation of why symptoms are being experienced coupled with reassurance that they are part of a normal cycle and not a disease process may help. Symptoms of fluid retention may be relieved by a thiazide diuretic; symptoms of anxiety may be helped by a mild tranquilliser; and headaches and other aches and pains may be relieved by simple analgesics. Any drugs given will excite a significant placebo response and vitamin B_6 may be used as a cheap, safe placebo. In severe cases not helped by simpler treatment, progesterone suppositories or pessaries (Cyclogest) are worth considering.

NB There is no doubt that premenstrual changes exist but their existence does not imply that they are due to disease or that they need treatment.

Psoriasis

Common skin disorder of unknown aetiology. It usually appears between the ages of 15 and 30 and shows different degrees of activity. Over a third of cases will remit, either spontaneously or after treatment, but the length of remission is variable.

Clinical diagnosis is generally easy. The classical lesion is a red, raised, scaly (white or silvery) plaque with sharply demarcated edges. Knees, elbows, sacrum and scalp are the most common sites. Pitted, hyperkeratotic or onycholytic nails may occur.

Patients should be told that psoriasis is: not contagious; not a sign of internal disease; not going to leave scars or marks when it clears; likely to remit (unpredictably); likely to be helped by sunshine. They should also understand that although treatment may improve the condition there is no permanent cure available. For those who want treatment, local applications of coal tar or dithranol preparations should be tried first. Topical steroids are indicated for new lesions, psoriasis in the groins, axillae and face, and for chronic plaques.

NB Although psoriasis cannot be cured the GP can still do a lot to help.

Raynaud's disease

In its mild form, this disease usually affects women. Digital artery spasm in cold weather makes the fingers go dead and white. After minutes or hours the circulation returns accompanied by pain and flushing of the affected fingers. There is no specific treatment. Cigarette smoking should be avoided and the hands kept as warm as possible at all times.

NB Raynaud's disease that is secondary to use of vibrating tools, collagen diseases, severe anaemia etc is a more serious condition.

Ringworm

Fungi are mostly transmitted from person to person though they may be acquired from cats, dogs and cattle.
   Ringworm of the groin (*Tinea cruris*) starts with erythema and maceration of the skin and spreads out in an annular pattern with a raised red scaly margin. Perspiration should be avoided as far as possible and topical preparations—e.g., Whitfield's ointment, clotrimazole (Canestan)—should be used. If inflammation is severe, hydrocortisone 1% may help. If lesions are chronic then oral griseofulvin 500 mg daily for one month may be needed.
   Ringworm of the body (*Tinea corporis*) characteristically forms a ring with an active edge and no clearing in the centre. Topical antifungals should be used but if infection does not clear griseofulvin may be needed.

NB Household pets may need to be checked by a vet.

Rubella

Rubella has an incubation period of 10–21 days before maculopapular rash, suboccipital lymphadenopathy and mild fever develop. Symptoms last 2–4 days and patients are infectious 5 days before and 5 days after the rash. Clinical diagnosis is notoriously inaccurate.
   Maternal rubella in pregnancy is associated with congenital abnormalities. If infection develops in the first 3–4 months of pregnancy then there is only a 1 in 3 chance of a completely normal child being born and termination should be considered.
   Presentation of a patient who fears she has contacted rubella in

early pregnancy is not uncommon. Pregnancy should be confirmed and rubella antibody titre estimated (over 80% of women of child-bearing age are immune). If there is no detectable rubella HI anti-body a second specimen should be taken 7–10 days after the onset of any rubella-like illness or 30 days after the last day of contact if no illness develops. Seroconversion indicates rubella.

If antibodies are detected in serum taken within 10 days of con-tact the patient can be regarded as immune. Antibodies detected in serum taken more than 10 days after contact may be from a developing or remote infection. A repeat titre is necessary and a rise would indicate current infection while a static low titre would exclude recent rubella.

NB Intrapractice screening and vaccination can eliminate the risk of congenital rubella.

Scabies

Highly contagious and most often acquired by sharing a bed with an infected person. There is often a positive family history. General-ised irritation when going to bed at night is usually the presenting symptom with a rash developing later. Burrows on the hands or deep, red papules on the buttocks or genitalia are diagnostic though by the time the patient presents there is also usually a generalised excoriated papular urticarial rash.

Treatment consists of two applications of benzyl benzoate lotion to all members of the affected household (gamma benzene hexach-loride in a 1% cream is preferable for children). The lotion must be applied to all the skin surface from the neck to the soles of the feet. The patient should be warned that irritation may well persist for 1–2 weeks after successful treatment and that genital papules may persist for months.

NB Suspect scabies in anyone whose itchy rash is worse at night.

Shingles

Like chickenpox, shingles is caused by the herpes zoster virus. Older people are generally affected and present with pain (often severe) felt unilaterally in the affected cutaneous segment. Between two and fourteen days later one or more blotchy red patches appear, to be followed in 24 hours by the characteristic vesicles. Vesicles may persist for up to 5 weeks and in 5% of cases will be followed by post-herpetic neuralgia.

Trigeminal involvement with its associated corneal ulceration and other eye complications demand ophthalmic management. Strong analgesics may be needed, though pain will be rapidly relieved by prednisolone, a short course of which will also help prevent post herpetic neuralgia.

NB Severe pain in the chest or abdomen occurring before the rash develops may cause diagnostic confusion.

Sinusitis

Most commonly affects the maxillary sinus. Clinical features include tenderness over the inflamed sinus, pus in the middle meatus and postnasal space, and some degree of constitutional upset.

Decongestants and analgesics help though antibiotics should be used sooner rather than later, particularly if frontal or ethmoidal sinuses seem to be involved.

NB Sinusitis may present as upper jaw toothache.

Soiling

Soiling or persisting diarrhoea in children demands a rectal examination as impacted faeces will often be found. Inital treatment with glycerine suppositories or Micralex enema should be followed by regular laxative use coupled with toilet training to try to resolve the problem.

NB Neither paediatricians nor child psychiatrists can easily help the encopretic child.

Sore throats

Caused by viruses in up to 80% of cases and clinical signs correlate poorly with the aetiological agent. Plenty of fluids and simple analgesics should be advised with penicillin best reserved for patients with a moderate degree of constitutional upset and no other symptoms suggestive of a viral upper respiratory tract infection. Throat swabs will rarely influence either management or outcome.

NB The worst-looking throats may well be glandular fever.

Snoring

Tends to have an adverse effect on everyone except the snorer. Kinking of the trachea by a sagging chin may be an aetiological factor and wearing a cervical collar (a rolled-up newspaper wrapped in a headscarf) at night might help.

NB If the worst comes to the worst earplugs may give some relief.

Squints

In babies, demand ophthalmic referral whenever mother or doctor suspect their presence. Negative examination does not exclude developing or intermittent squints.

Squints developing for the first time in older children or adults will cause diplopia (relieved by covering the squinting eye). A cause should be diligently sought.

NB Babies with broad epicanthic folds are as likely to have squints as other babies.

Sticky eyes

Developing within a few days of birth, sticky eyes should be swabbed before being treated with an antibiotic ointment. Recurrence or non-resolution should raise the question of chlamydia infection. Special culture will be required and if positive the baby may be treated with oral erythromycin.

A blocked nasolachryimal duct may contribute to the infection. Mother should be taught how to massage the duct upwards towards the inner canthus so that stasis in the upper blind end is reduced. Patency may well not be achieved until 6–9 months of age and referral for probing should certainly not be before this time.

NB Reassurance that sticky eyes pose no threat to eyesight helps Mother to cope with recurrences.

Styes

Localised infections of the glands of the lid margin. After a few days of painful swelling a bead of pus will be discharged and resolution will take place.

No treatment is necessary though antibiotic ointment may prevent emerging staphylococci from infecting another lash follicle.

NB Recurrent styes are not a sign of being 'run down'.

Sunburn

Fairly common self-inflicted injury. Initial erythema occurs during exposure and disappears shortly afterwards. Delayed erythema, accompanied by pain and discomfort, begins about 3 hours after exposure and persists for about 48 hours. Peeling follows erythema.

Mild cases need use nothing more than a soothing cream four times a day but severer cases may need to take simple analgesics and apply a topical steroid cream for 2–3 days to decrease the inflammatory response.

NB All cases should avoid further injudicious exposure to sunlight.

Teething

Occurs from 6 months to 6 years and may cause some pain, irritability and excess salivation. Although a useful excuse for crying and sleeping difficulties the diagnosis should not be made until general conditions have been excluded.

No treatment is necessary other than paracetamol elixir for pain.

NB Painful gums may cause hard items of food to be refused.

Tenosynovitis

An inflammatory condition of tendon sheaths which produces pain that is worse during movement of the tendon. Localised tenderness, swelling and crepitus may be present and treatment may be with a short course of a non-steroidal anti-inflammatory drug coupled with a tubigrip bandage to help decrease movement of the affected part.

NB This is mostly an isolated condition not associated with systemic disease.

Tennis elbow

Can affect anyone and produces severe pain on the outer side of the arm especially with movements requiring the hand to be turned on its palm. There is localised tenderness over or just below the lateral epicondyle and symptoms will wax and wane until naturally resolving after about 2 years.

A local anaesthetic/steroid injection at the site of maximum tenderness, repeated if necessary one month later, will cure 60% of patients.

NB Medial epicondylitis is known as golfer's elbow.

Threadworms

These live in the bowel in up to 40% of under-10-year-olds. Pruritus ani (particularly nocturnal) is the only symptom that they produce, apart from anxiety if an adult worm is seen in the stool. Faecal-oral spread by scratching fingers causes reinfection of the host and new infections in the rest of the family.

As worms live for only 6–8 weeks strict family hygiene for that length of time will resolve the infection. Hygiene advice should be given: affected child should have nails cut short, wear pyjamas and possibly gloves to bed, bathe each morning carefully washing perianal skin, use own towel, change and wash clothes and bedclothes. In addition all the family should have a strict toilet hygiene. Advice may be coupled with a prescription for a piperazine compound—e.g. Pripsen to be taken in 2 doses one week apart. All members of the family should be treated at the same time, but each should be given an individual prescription.

NB Prescription without hygiene advice will result in recurrence.

Tinnitus

May be aggravating and distressing. Noises are loudest when the environment is quietest. Wax is the only likely remediable cause as most cases are due to inner ear problems associated with increased age. Most patients are deaf to some degree and their tinnitus will be a persistent problem which no treatment will help.

NB Other noises can be used to mask out the tinnitus—e.g. keeping a radio on may help a sufferer to get off to sleep.

Toothache

Usually presents when dentists are not available or feared. If no infection is present then advice about suitable analgesics is all that is necessary. If tooth or gum infection exists then penicillin V or erythromycin should be prescribed. In all cases a dental appointment should be advised.

NB Earache without any other signs of ear disease is often due to pain referred from teeth.

Umbilical hernia

Varies in size and is common in young babies. Soft and easily reduced with virtually no risk of strangulation. Disappears spontaneously as the baby grows and requires no treatment of any sort.

NB Parents should understand that the hernia will appear when the baby cries, not that the baby is crying because the hernia has appeared.

Undescended testicles

Found in 1 in 5 premature and 1 in 25 full-term boys. Most will descend spontaneously by the age of 1 year but if they are not in the scrotum by then orchidopexy is indicated. Operation is probably best carried out between 1 and 2 years and certainly before the age of 5.

NB A cold surgery or cold hands will activate the cremaster reflex and make examination unreliable.

Varicose veins

Present, to some degree, in 2 out of 3 adults. Most cases present because of the patient's dissatisfaction with their cosmetic appearance. Aching on standing with heavy, painful and swollen legs may occur as may complications of impaired skin nutrition such as eczema or pigmentation and varicose ulceration.

Diagnosis is straightforward. Clinical localisation of incompetent perforating veins is highly inaccurate.

Most cases require no specific treatment. General advice should be given—namely, high roughage diet, keep active, avoid sitting or standing in the same position for any length of time, avoid crossing the legs while sitting. Elastic support stockings (full length, standard circular yarn type with no toes) worn regularly will give relief and clinical improvement whether surgical treatment is contemplated or not.

Injection of sclerosing agents is associated with recurrence in 65% of cases after 6 years. With surgery about 25% of patients will need further treatment after 5 years.

NB Varicose veins are not a contraindication to the pill.

Varicose ulcers

Develop in about 3% of patients with varicose veins especially those with a history of deep vein thrombosis. Ulceration usually occurs in the region of the ankle just above or below the malleoli and may arise spontaneously or after minor injury or infection. Varicose ulcers cause little pain but if present can be relieved by raising the foot.

Treatment is long drawn-out and both the ulcer and the underlying swelling and congestion of the skin need to be dealt with. Raising the leg, with the patient lying flat, followed by compression bandaging is essential for healing. In some cases prolonged bed rest may be needed. A good diet is also essential.

A considerable variety of paste bandages may be used as may Debrisan in resistant cases. Your trainer is likely to have his own favourite treatment.

NB The practice nurse is likely to be more knowledgeable about the management of this condition than you. Do not be afraid to seek her advice or refer patients to her.

Verrucas

These are warts on the feet. Pressure may make them painful on walking. They may be distinguished from simple corns by the presence of blood vessels (paring of the surface of a wart will reveal minute bleeding points).

If they are producing unacceptable pain or deformity, treatment may be indicated. Salicyclic acid collodion solution or plasters may be used as may formaldehyde gel (Veracur).

NB Verrucas are no bar to swimming. If misdirected official bans exist then wearing a waterproof plaster while at the pool will get round them.

Warts

Generally present for cosmetic reasons because they are only painful if they become secondarily infected or are being traumatised. Before any treatment is undertaken the following factors must be considered: warts naturally resolve (within months in children); there is no drug effective against the wart virus so treatment is empirical; most treatments have poorer results than if the wart is left alone; treatment may be painful while the wart is usually painless; a naturally resolving wart leaves no scars while a badly treated one might; if natural immunity has not developed to the wart virus then a high relapse rate is to be expected.

Most cases need only explanation of the natural history or, if the parents insist on treatment, advice to buy a simple remedy from the chemist and do the work themselves. A few warts causing pain or deformity may need to be removed and if painting with 10% salicylic acid collodion BPC twice daily for 2–3 months does not effect an improvement referral for cautery or cryotherapy may be indicated.

NB There is no particular reason for doctors to be concerned in the management of this benign lesion and a well-briefed practice nurse should be able to cope with most cases.

Wax in the ears

May accumulate to occlude the meatus and produce deafness, tinnitus or even vertigo. Provided that the ear is not too painful and that there is no suggestion of perforation of the tympanic membrane syringing is the treatment of choice. If wax is hard then the use of olive oil or drops such as Cerumol four times a day for 3 days before syringing will make the task easier. The patient can buy these drops before coming to the nurse or doctor for syringing.

NB The wax in babies' ears is very soft and may present as 'a runny ear'.

Whooping cough

Has an incubation period of 7–10 days before the catarrhal phase, which resembles a severe cold, begins. Instead of resolving in 3–4 days fever persists and coughing increases, beginning to occur in bouts and being most prominent at night. After 2 weeks the paroxysmal phase with its characteristic paroxysms followed by vomiting and in many cases whooping, develops and persists for another 3–4 weeks before the child will get better. Infectivity is highest during the catarrhal phase (when the diagnosis is most difficult) and persists for about 4 weeks in all.

No antispasmodic or cough medicine has been shown to affect the cough though an antihistamine, given at night for its sedative effect, may be helpful as, alternatively, might elixir diazepam. A warm humid atmosphere will help relieve coughing spasms and meals are best kept small and frequent if vomiting is troublesome. Although there is little evidence that they help, antibiotics (erythromycin or amoxycillin) are likely to be prescribed at some stage.

Most severe cases tend to occur in children below the age of 6 months and the mainstay of treatment is constant supervision and careful nursing. if paroxysms are severe, social circumstances poor or complications develop then hospital admission is indicated.

NB Prevention by vaccination is far superior to the largely ineffectual treatment we have to offer established cases.

Wry-neck

Wry-neck or acute torticollis due to muscular spasm from viral myalgia or secondary to infected cervical glands is slow in onset with a tender muscle found on examination. Treatment consists of rest in a collar, prescription or advice about suitable analgesia and an antibiotic if adenitis is present.

Joint dysfunction causing wry-neck is sudden in onset with

severe pain provoked by neck movement. Traction may give quick relief. Stand behind patient who is seated on low stool; put one hand under the chin and the other under the occiput; pull steadily upwards while keeping the neck straight; if pain is worsened—*stop*—but if improved then repeat several times before putting on collar and giving suitable analgesia.

NB a cervical collar helps to rest the acutely painful neck and in an emergency can be made by rolling a newspaper to make a flat band wide enough to immobilise the neck when placed round it like a parson's collar and held in place with a scarf.

16. LONG-TERM PROBLEMS

Certain diseases need long-term treatment and careful supervision if serious disability is to be kept to a minimum. The most important ones are as follows:

diabetes	rheumatoid arthritis
hypertension	chronic bronchitis
asthma	peptic ulcer
epilepsy	ulcerative colitis and Crohn's disease
thyroid disease	pernicious anaemia

Diabetes, hypertension and asthma are discussed in greater detail later in this chapter. There are other chronic diseases, such as multiple sclerosis, where medical intervention has little influence on the clinical course but is important for maintaining mobility and the morale of the patient and his family. Complications may arise from the disease process itself, from the drugs used in treatment, from concurrent illness or incompatible medication, or from the lifestyle of the patient. It may be possible to influence all of these.

To be successful, a plan of care has to be drawn up for each patient individually. Even more than for short-term illness, the patient has to share the doctor's enthusiasm for the treatment and work in partnership with the doctor, if it is to be carried out effectively. After all, for a patient living in the community it is not the doctor who treats the patient but the patient who treats himself with the doctor's help. It is therefore a waste of time for the doctor to try to impose a pattern of care with which the patient is unable or unwilling to cooperate.

When plan is first drawn up, the following areas have to be considered.

Information

The patient should plan to learn as much as he wants and is capable of understanding about the disease, its probable course, the problems that may arise, the method, purpose, importance and side effects of treatment, the importance of regular visits to the surgery and what events should lead him to seek advice between routine visits. The GP, perhaps in cooperation with other members of the primary health care team, is likely to be the main source of information. It is not necessary or desirable for all information to be presented at once. Information is more likely to be understood and retained if it is presented piecemeal over several visits and in response to questions from the patient. Much of it will have to be repeated on several occasions.

Providing time for questions from the patient is of the utmost importance. It cannot be assumed that he will ask anything he wants to know without prompting or that, if he has been in hospital, he already has all the information he needs. Leaflets about individual diseases can be very useful and there are some excellent ones produced by pharmaceutical companies. Societes such as the British Diabetic Association are also useful sources of information as well as of moral support.

Details of Management

Drug dosage should be kept as simple as possible, even at the cost of some loss of effectiveness. It is better to take a single daily dose of a long-acting or slow-release preparation regularly than divided doses of a short-acting one erratically. If the patient is to regulate his own dosage, as in diabetes or asthma, he must understand how the drug acts and what changes he should feel free to make. Many asthmatics fail to derive benefit from even regular use of sodium cromoglycate because their bouts of exercise, or exposure to allergens, occur long after the previous dose. For instance, a child using his Spinhaler conscientiously at 7 am, 12 noon, 5 pm, and 10 pm will still develop asthma during his physical education lesson at 11 am or football after school at 4 pm. Even a stable diabetic may go into hypoglycaemic coma every Saturday afternoon after the football match, if he is unable to reduce his insulin for the occasion as well as increasing his calorie intake.

For some drugs the technique of administration is of crucial importance. This is obvious in the case of insulin, but it is also essential in the use of inhalers. Patients should be taught to use inhalers and observed using them from time to time. Some people find powdery inhalants extremely unpleasant but may not tell the doctor so unless specifically asked. They may use a pressurised alternative—or electric nebuliser—more regularly.

It is important that the patient knows what to expect from a drug. many hypertensive patients stop taking the tablets because they do not 'feel any better on them' just as asthmatics may give up sodium cromoglycate because it does not relieve the bronchospasm.

Obtaining repeat prescriptions should be as trouble-free as possible. To save frequent visits to the surgery there is no reason why a patient on long-term treatment should not receive three months' supply at a time or postdated prescriptions.

Arrangements for Follow-up

The question of whom to see, for what and when will vary with the disease, the patient, the available facilities and on whether the care is being shared with a hospital outpatient department. Some conditions, such as diabetes, are sufficiently common and complex to warrant a special clinic where a nurse can work alongside the doctor, preparing the patient for clinical examination and carrying out certain procedures—such as weight, blood pressure, urine and blood testing. Some doctors may prefer the patient to have the blood test a few days before a visit so that the result is available at the clinic. Some patients may be unable or unwilling to attend such a clinic. Ideally, arrangements should be as flexible as possible.

The biggest difficulty in general practice is ensuring that the patient attends for follow-up. Special arrangements have to be made for this. Most doctors would feel that it is not enough to leave it to the patient unless the patient knows all that the doctor does about the possible consequences of inadequate care. This is unlikely to be the case and so it remains the doctor's responsibility.

Diabetes

Treatment for diabetes is likely to be initiated in hospital in insulin-dependent diabetics, by the GP for the rest.

Information

Techniques of urine or blood testing and insulin administration are usually taught by nursing staff. It is important for doctors to know what the patient is being taught.

Useful tip: Disposable syringes may be used repeatedly if kept for the same patient. They are not yet available on prescription but are not expensive to buy. The district nurse is helpful in checking on techniques and giving injections for blind or disabled.

Understanding. The patient should understand:

- What a hypoglycaemic attack is like, what causes it and what to do both at once and to avoid another.
- The interrelation between diet, activity and insulin dosage.
- What to do if ill.
- When to seek urgent help—e.g. for vomiting.
- The importance of conscientious control.
- Care of the skin and feet.

Information for relatives. It is especially important for the family to know how to recognise the beginning of a hypoglycaemia coma—e.g. by irritability or irrational behaviour—and what to do.

British Diabetic Association. The patient should be given details of the association.

Details of management

A cooperation card or booklet for the patient to carry is extremely useful. One is produced free by Hoechst.

Diet

Details of diet should include amounts of carbohydrate or equivalent proteins or fats. Must be simple and understood and agreed by both patient and doctor. May need to be adjusted according to weight.

156

Food must be eaten regularly in reasonable amounts. Insulin-dependent diabetics usually cooperate well with this but many of the others have a single large meal a day, making control impossible. All diabetics should carry emergency food.

Urine or blood testing

It is better to do random testing occasionally at different times of the day than test sample at same time every day.

Insulin dosage

Dosage should be written down by doctor in booklet or cooperation card and should include type, strength, number of marks on syringe and number of units to be given.

Activity

Diabetics should be encouraged to lead as normal a life as possible.

Lifestyle

- Regular eating habits are obviously very important.
- Diabetics are at greater risk from smoking than non-diabetics.
- Contraception may pose problems. The pill carries an increased risk in diabetics and the intrauterine contraceptive device is reputed to be less effective than in other women.
- Pregnancy is particularly hazardous. Control by frequent blood glucose measurements by patient improves prognosis.

Arrangements for follow-up

Stable diabetic patients without complications may be cared for by their GP alone, but if care is shared with a hospital clinic it should be clearly understood who does what, or important elements of care may be omitted.

Regular routine visits are essential, the frequency depending on the stability and quality of control achieved by the patient.

All diabetics should be seen at least once every six months.

Suggested plan for routine care of diabetes without complications

Every visit (6 months)

Examine interval blood sugar; weight; review patient's tests, well being, symptoms and ask if there are any queries.

Once a year

Test mid-stream urine specimen, take blood pressure and examine feet. Examination of fundi after short-acting mydriatic.

Every two years

Full central nervous system examination.

Hypertension

Diagnosis

This may be made during screening programme, or at routine examination for hospital admission, employment or life insurance. At least three readings should be taken on separate occasions before drug treatment is initiated. Usual to treat persistent levels of over 150/100 in the young; older people only if symptoms or signs present, e.g. angina, breathlessness, cardiomegaly, retinopathy.

Investigation and treatment

In straightforward cases this is normally carried out by the GP; shared care with consultant physician in complicated ones.

Information

Leaflets are produced free by some drug companies. Patients needs to know

(1) as much as possible about the disease, its natural history and the importance of treatment;
(2) the importance of life style and how to cope with stress, (e.g. relaxation exercises);

(3) how to lose weight and stop smoking;
(4) how to take the drugs.

Details of management

A cooperation card is useful.

Diet

Reduce weight if necessary and then maintain ideal weight. Low animal fats probably sensible, important if lipoproteins abnormal.

Lifestyle

- Recognise stressful factors and avoid or learn to deal with them.
- Practise relaxation—20 minutes twice a day if possible and when under stress.
- Regular exercise.
- Stop smoking.
- Contraception and pregnancy need care.

Drugs

Dose should be written in cooperation card.

Follow-up

Regular and indefinite (although it may be possible to phase out treatment in some people after a few years).

Arrangements for follow-up

If care is shared with hospital, it should be clearly understood who does what and when. Some sort of recall system is necessary, e.g. card index or computer.

Visits have to be frequent at first (e.g. every two weeks) until dosage is adjusted to produce desired result. After that, three-monthly or, in stable cases, six-monthly visits only may be needed.

Suggested plan for routine care of hypertensives without complications

(Can be shared between doctor and nurse.)

Every visit

- General inquiry about wellbeing, problems, lifestyle.
- Blood pressure.
- Weight.
- Confirmation of drug regimen.

Every 2 years. Blood urea and electrolytes.
Every 5 years. Chest x-ray; ECG; examine fundi.

Asthma

Diagnosis

Asthma is often missed as chest clear when patient seen; suspect children with nocturnal cough or coughing and breathlessness after exercise. Useful to be able to exercise patient in or around the surgery.

Information

Success of management depends entirely on how well the patient uses the advice and drugs he is given. The patient needs:

(1) To know as much as possible about the disease and its management. Excellent booklets available from Fison's.
(2) To recognise trigger factors and avoid them if possible (e.g. household pets) or take sodium cromoglycate before exposure.
(3) To understand how and when to use drugs—especially the difference between prophylaxis (e.g. sodium cromoglycate) and treatment (e.g. salbutamol).
(4) To learn technique of using inhaler: pressurised inhalers are frequently misused.
(5) To lead as normal a life as possible.
(6) To recognise danger signals when an acute attack fails to respond to treatment.

Relatives need to understand the disease and its management, especially if the patient is a child. A balance must be found between neglect and overcaution.

Details of management

It may be useful for the patient, for short periods, to keep a chart of symptoms and treatment—these are available in the Fison's booklet.

Diet

Obesity should be avoided.

Exercise

Regular, protected by sodium cromoglycate if necessary.

Lifestyle

No smoking at all, ever. Emotional stress may be an important trigger factor. May have to avoid polluted atmospheres and allergens (e.g. animals).

Drugs

Aspirin precipitates asthma in some subjects; β blockers should be avoided.

- Have emergency plan for acute attacks; e.g. call doctor, go straight to hospital.
- If a short course of systemic steroids is needed, the daily dose should be written down.
- If the patient has own peak flow meter, he may telephone doctor to report readings.
- Every patient should be observed using an inhaler to check that it is being used correctly.

Arrangements for follow-up

Most symptomatic asthmatics are easy to follow up because they ask for prescriptions. Some, especially children, may have persistent or repeated mild asthma and do not request treatment. Recall system advisable especially for the young.

Frequency depends upon severity, whether seasonal and upon how much the patient can be relied upon to carry out the treatment correctly.

Suggested plan for routine care of young asthmatic (not taking steroids)

Every visit (3–6 months)

- General inquiry about wellbeing, exercise, tolerance, frequency and severity of symptoms, detailed drug usage.

NB watch for those whose activities are limited unnecessarily because of asthma).

- Peak flow measurement
- Height and weight
- Review medication and check that it is being used correctly.

PART III
CHOOSING A PRACTICE

17. THE PRACTICE

The number of practice vacancies available each year are fewer than the number of vocationally trained job seekers. Viewed as a complex game of musical chairs your objective, when the music stops, is to be occupying not just any job but one which you are reasonably sure is going to fulfil your personal and professional needs. Life-long partnerships are being formed and mistakes can be costly both financially and in terms of morale.

For some, chance will provide a good practice with little effort. For the majority, a great deal of thought, care and hard work will be necessary before a reasonable partnership is gained.

Decide What You Want

Before looking for a practice you must have a fairly clear idea of what you are looking for. It is worth taking time to draw a pen picture of your ideal practice noting which features are essential as opposed to desirable, and which are tolerable rather than intolerable. The more realistic you are in your expectations the better, and the less restrictive your conditions are then the more choice you will have.

While personal or family reasons may limit your choice, the following are some general points to consider.

Practice location

The more popular the area the more competition there will be for the job and the lower the likely initial financial rewards.

Find out the availability and cost of housing (lowest in north-east of England), and standard of local primary and secondary schools.

Consider the proximity, or otherwise, to relatives, and scope for pursuing outside interests.

Practice size

Ask how many doctors, there are in practice, and the number of patients on list (East Midlands offers largest average lists, 2371; Scotland lowest, 1856).

Ask about staff: practice manager; practice nurses; attached health visitors; community nurses, etc.

Practice workload

Consider population characteristics, e.g. highest morbidity and mortality in Wales, lowest in South-east England, holday areas have increased work in the summer; over 65s and below 5s are heaviest users of medical care. Also:

- Is work, including out of hours cover, shared equally?
- What use is made of deputising services, rotas with other practices?
- Is there an appointment system?
- What use is made of ancillary staff to cope with workload?
- Is there extra practice work, e.g., clinical assistantships; GP hospitals or maternity units; factory work?
- Is the practice on top of its work or is the work on top of it?
- Find out about annual holidays/study leave (on average 6–8 weeks in all).

Practice premises

Consider the following:

- If it is a DHA health centre no capital will be required by new partner.
- If private premises, can you affored a share of the capital assets (£25 000 on average)?
- If dispensing, is capital needed for drug stocks?
- Does each doctor have his own room?
- Is there a library; doctors' meeting room; treatment room etc.?
- What is the standard of equipment and furnishing?
- What is the standard of records; age/sex register; computer?
- Is there any possibility of future alterations/improvement?

Partners

You will need to know something about your partners;

(1) What are their ages; sex; political/religious views; interests?

(2) Do they get on well with each other and will you be able to get on well with them?

(3) Are they flexible enough to accept changes if a good case is put forward for them?

(4) Are their wives involved in the practice and if so will yours have to be?

(5) If they are not teaching or doing research themselves would they cooperate with someone who wanted to be doing these.

Potential income

- How much work for how much money?
- Initial salary (usually for first 6 months)?
- How long to parity (averages 2–3 years but quicker in less desirable areas or where parity is low anyway) and what shares until it is reached?
- Is all income shared equally and, if not, how exactly is it divided up?

Look at the Options

About a year before you want your practice start reading the job columns of the *British Medical Journal* (*BMJ*). Take a note of any jobs that particularly interest you so that in about 4–6 months' time, when you will be applying, you can see if any of them come up again. If so, is it a new vacancy or has someone left after only a few months? If they did not appoint anyone is it because they were choosy or are there problems in the practice?

Use various sources for job information.

The local grapevine

Your trainer or course organiser may well be approached by or know of practices that are looking for new partners. He may also advertise your availability by word of mouth and gain you an exclusive interview to a possible partnership.

Working in different practices during your trainee year not only helps you to decide your own priorities for practice but also increases your local contacts, any one of whom might recommend you to a colleague who is looking for a partner.

The British Medical Association

The Personal Services Bureau of the British Medical Association (BMA) provides a comprehensive service to members. Detailed descriptions of practice vacancies may be obtained from them. It is worth getting the details of several practices both to see what variety exists and what financial conditions prevail in areas you are interested in. Remember that they may have details of vacancies not advertised in the *BMJ*.

Advertisements

The *BMJ* is the best sourse and few jobs will not be advertised in it at some stage. Many, however, may be readvertised or even advertised for the first time in free medical newspapers such as *Pulse, General Practitioner* and *Riker*.

Carefully-worded informative advertisements can tell you a lot about a practice. One-line-ads with box numbers tell you even more. Remember to be a little cynical when reading about any practice and read between the lines, e.g. 'ample time for outside interests' often implies little money to spend on them; 'equal work for equal money' may mean that parity is low because all the other partners keep their incomes from outside the practice.

Family Practitioner Committees

If one area interests you then an approach to the Family Practitioners Committee (FPC) administrator may be worthwhile. At best he may know of a practice vacancy, at worst he can keep your name and address and pass it on to any practice that seeks his advice on taking on a new partner.

Self-advertising

If one particular area especially attracts you then a detailed advertisement about yourself in the *BMJ* might just marry you up with a practice in the area which had not got around to advertising itself.

Start applying

Most practices are looking for potential partners who can start work fairly soon and jobs mainly tend not to be available for more than 6 months. That, then, is the best time scale for applying.

Once you have spotted interesting advertisements make sure that you fulfil the requirements that they stipulate. Then decide whether you want any more information before going ahead with a formal application. If you decide to go ahead either write, telephone (it is helpful to get a general impression of how you are dealt with) or even visit the practice to clarify any details you think important. The further information may put you off and save you the trouble of applying formally.

When you have made up your mind to apply compile an easily understood well-typed *curriculum vitae* giving all the relevant information about you without being unduly detailed or boastful. Make sure you include some family background and social information as well as the usual medical information. If you are quoting potential referees (your trainer should be one; the local course organiser, or a local consultant with whom you have worked closely, might be the other) seek their permission first and, as a point of courtesy, keep them informed of your progress. Always include a short, handwritten, covering letter indicating what particular features of the practice have attracted you. Good handwriting will help your application.

Remember that it is not unusual for there to be 70 or more applicants for a job, so your aim is to be one of the few selected for interview. You must therefore sell yourself by ensuring that your application is as attractively presented as possible. No matter how much you have to offer, if you apply in a different or offhand way you will not get the chance to show it.

Finally, resist the natural tendency to expect to get the job you have applied for—this means you will leave other possible jobs to hang fire. Apply for all those that interest you, even if it means two or three at a time. After all, who can tell what is going to happen?

The interview

If you are asked to come for an interview the likelihood is that you will have to do better than, probably, between two and five short-listed rivals before you can consider the job yours. You may all be interviewed on the same day or asked to come individually to spend

169

a day at the practice meeting everyone in an informal and leisurely fashion. Spouses may also be invited but, if not, married doctors should ensure that their spouses see round the practice and meet the partners before any final decisions are made. At an interview your aim is to make as good an impression as possible while assessing your potential partners just as carefully as they are assessing you.

Dress conventionally and smartly; turn up a little early; be polite to everyone you meet; talk intelligently and intelligibly while trying to put the interviewers at their ease; be confident but not boring or boastful; above all, appear interested in what you are being asked even if the point of a question escapes you. The questions that you are asked are unlikely to fall into any predictable pattern and are best dealt with spontaneously. The questions you ask should be carefully prepared and should be friendly, interested and reasonably enthusiastic without being in any way critical. As much can be learned by the quality of your questions as by the quality of your answers.

Partnership is based on mutual trust, respect and esteem and the key factor is compatibility. If partners like each other and get on well together no problem remains a problem for long; if they do not, life will quickly become intolerable.

If you have been shown kindness or been entertained by some of the partners write and thank them or their wives after the interview. Good manners cost nothing, whether you are going to get the job or not.

Most practices expect to pay interviewees' expenses.

The Partnership Offer

A successful interview may be followed by an offer, but usually a further more leisurely meeting will take place before the offer is either made or confirmed. Despite having come so far, if you are dubious about any aspects of the practice keep asking until you get satisfactory answers. It is dangerous to gloss over problems, whatever pressure you may feel to accept the job and secure your future.

Now is the time to discuss practice finance in detail. From the advertisement, or before interview, you will have gained a rough idea of parity and the terms on offer. If they were not generally acceptable you should not have come this far. To emphasise financial aspects overmuch during the selection process is probably unwise but to discuss them carefully afterwards is estimable prudence.

If the initial practice details stated categorically the financial terms on offer then there is really no negotiating to do. If, however, the time to parity and shares have been left open for discussion your knowledge of what is on offer elsewhere is vital. Broadly speaking, the minimum acceptable salary for the first 6 months to a year would be equivalent to your VTA + car allowance. A share giving a higher net (after-practice expenses) income than this should follow, rising in equal stages to parity in 2–3 years.

Make sure you know if working capital is needed. If a share of the premises has to be purchased then the property must be professionally valued and finance sought from a bank or an equally cheap source. The practice accounts must be seen and examined and advice should be taken from the practice accountant, bank manager and solicitor. One point that should be brought to the accountant's attention is the situation that prevails if the partnership, on your joining, elects to remain the same for tax purposes. Broadly speaking, this continuation election will mean extra tax for a newcomer and less tax for the incumbents. The accountant can, with the agreement of the partners, make sure that you suffer no financial loss from this device.

Read the partnership agreement carefully (it is well worth sending it to the BMA for their comments on its contents) and once all points are agreed have it drawn up again by the solicitor for everyone's protection. In addition to this have your final agreed offer given to you in writing.

Finally, during all this process you should have been keen and happy, but should not have altered your whole pattern of behaviour or practice to impress people. At some stage the mask would slip and problems could then arise. Remember most partnerships will accept a newcomer with the proviso that either party can withdraw from the agreement within the first 6 months if things do not seem to be working out.

INDEX

177

Mumps

Incubation 18-21 days

Infection 2-3/7 before swelling → until
glands d.l.

Measles

Incubation 10-14⁺ days

Infection 5/7 before rash → 5/7 after
temp↓ a rash gone.

Chickenpox

Incubation 14-21 days

Infection 1/7 before rash → 6/7 after rash
ie. vesicles all crusted.

Post vacc Pyrexia –

2/12 old FT babe – 40mg paracet
ie 1.7ml of
120g/5.0

2/12 preterm infant → 10mg/kg.